A VIRUS OF LOVE
& Other Tales of Medical Detection

A VIRUS OF LOVE

& OTHER TALES OF MEDICAL DETECTION

Charles T. Gregg

University of New Mexico
Albuquerque

Library of Congress Cataloging in Publication Data
Gregg, Charles T.
  A virus of love and other tales of medical detection.

  Originally published: New York: Scribner, c1983.
  Includes bibliographical references and index.
  1. Diseases—Causes and theories of causation—
Miscellanea.   I. Title.
RB151.G74   1985   616.07   84–17204
ISBN 0-8263-0793-0 (pbk.)

For Beth, with profound admiration
for her dignity and courage

Acknowledgments

The quality of this book owes much to my friends, colleagues, and editors who have tried to persuade me to eliminate errors, inconsistencies, and bad jokes that grated on everyone's sensibilities except my own. That they frequently succeeded will be apparent; that they sometimes failed to persuade me to listen to reason will be clear as well. For those remaining errors and infelicities I am solely responsible.

Each of the following read the entire manuscript, in one of its several "final" versions, and made valuable suggestions: Ernest C. Anderson, Ph.D., formerly Scientific Advisor to the Life Science Division of the University of California's Los Alamos National Laboratory (LANL); T. H. Chen, M.D., the University of California, Berkeley; and Walter R. Dowdle, Ph.D., Director of the Center for Infectious Disease, The Centers for Disease Control, Atlanta, Georgia. Their contributions, individually and collectively, were of inestimable value to me.

Susanne Kirk, Senior Editor at Charles Scribner's Sons, agreed to edit this book even though she had edited my previous book and cannot have forgotten the battles we fought over it. She may have hoped that the passage of a few years had made me less combative; if so I fear she was disappointed. Elizabeth Rapoport, Assistant Editor, brought to the project a sound scientific background, a vivid intelligence, and an amazing maturity for someone just a few months out of Yale. I consider myself most fortunate to have had such charming and competent editorial help; I'm a far better writer because of it.

Finally, my wife was unfailingly cheerful, supportive, and uncomplaining throughout the many months during which I was trying to write this book and fulfill my other professional responsibilities, to the virtual exclusion of vacations, parties, movies, concerts, travel, or walks in the forest. I owe her more than I can tell.

Contents

Without the Camp

I

The elderly man watched with grave dignity as I ran my fingers lightly over the mottled skin of his right forearm. To my inexpert touch his skin seemed dry, scaly, and possibly thickened, but I couldn't feel lumps under it that I thought might be there. Not that it mattered. His face and ears were covered with the distinctive nodules of lepromatous (or cutaneous) leprosy. He was the first case I'd ever seen.

II

A monk of the island monastery of Lindisfarne, off the North Sea coast of England, looked out to sea, then called excitedly to his fellows. Out of the mist, that June morning in A.D. 793, shot low, black ships propelled by broad, red sails and leaping banks of oars.

The chatter of the excited monks became murmurs of apprehension, then screams of pain and terror as the vessels drove up on the beach and giant, bearded men leaped howling from the bows brandishing battleaxes, swords, and spears. Shortly after, most of the monks were dead, the monastery buildings were in flames, and the Viking raiders were cheerfully loading their ships with Christian gold, silver, and tapestries for the short voyage home.

These sporadic raids continued for some eighty years before a mighty fleet of a hundred ships and a thousand Viking warriors under Ivar the Boneless landed on the North Sea beaches for a more extensive stay. The Norsemen surged to and fro across England for months, burning, raping, looting, and deposing and murdering kings, before their vessels returned to Scandinavia with slaves and riches. The Vikings continued to ravage England at their whim for more than two centuries.

Many Vikings came from Norway, whose sparse and rock-strewn soil could not feed her sons. It was to those icy fiords that many of the dragon ships returned with booty and, most important for this story, with slaves from England and Ireland. With those slaves and their Viking captors came leprosy to Norway; a millennium later, it passed to Minnesota, Michigan, the Dakotas, and Iowa with their descendants.

III

The Mexican woman was asleep before an open window, the blue of her nightgown matching the azure sky glimpsed occasionally through the fog swirling over the San Francisco hills. Although she was forty years old, her face was as fresh and unlined as a child's. Infiltration of the leprosy bacillus under her skin smoothed the faint wrinkles and lines she might otherwise have had; it had also destroyed her eyebrows. *Lepra bonita*—pretty leprosy—was first found in Mexico. Untreated, the woman wouldn't have been pretty much longer.

IV

Imagine yourself, for a moment, as a pretty Norwegian girl living in a small village at the edge of a fiord near Bergen in the fifteenth century. You expected soon to marry one of the strong young men of the village. But now you are being led to a small boat by your father and oldest brother, whose callused hands grip your elbows. Weeping, you are put into the boat, a small cloth with your few belongings is put in with you, and your father and brother shove the boat into the water. You are alone. Your boat is towed behind another rowed by four men.

Hours later the boat is pushed ashore at the edge of Byfiord beyond the village of Bergen, and one of the men gestures at a path leading up the bank. As you trudge upward, in tears again, you look back to see the men filling your boat with twigs and berries that they will burn to purify it before they return to the village.

At the top of the bank there is a rough wall with a gate. You knock. The gate opens. You drop your bundle and clasp both hands over your mouth to hold in a scream. The man who opened the gate is not old; there is no gray in his black hair. But most of his nose and part of his upper lip have rotted away. Saliva runs constantly from the triangular hole that is now his mouth and over his drooping lower lip; under his half-closed lids his eyes are an opaque white. "Welcome," he says in a hoarse voice, as an elderly woman whose face is a wasteland of bumps and nodules smiles a twisted greeting and picks up your small bundle.

You look numbly about the courtyard. Beside the well sits a man on whose leg is a sore so deep that you can see the bones, white and glistening, yet he contentedly smokes his pipe in the afternoon sun. Beside him a woman writhes in torment on the ground, her mouth forming screams that make no sound, for she has no voice. Another man, your father's age, sits leaning against the wall. He has neither fingers nor toes. He, too, is blind. Tears run constantly from his sightless eyes and make grotesque spots on his woolen shirt. Suddenly you know—what they are you will become! You turn to run, meaning to throw yourself into the fiord, but the gate has been shut and barred.

V

I greet the young Chicano in my rudimentary Spanish, "Buenas dias, coma esta?" As we shake hands, I notice that the third finger of his left hand, although it still has a distorted nail, is much shorter than the others. My guide, Dr. Robert Gelbar, points out a healed sore on the young man's arm. On his heel is another nearly healed ulcer as big as a quarter. This man is without feeling in his hands or feet. If a shoe pinches or a nail pierces his flesh, he will go on wearing the shoe until he or someone else notices the wound, which by then may be badly infected. The shortened finger is consequent to an injury, unnoticed at the time, followed by an infection that caused the bone to dissolve and be resorbed into the flesh around it. The fingers and toes of leprosy victims don't fall off. Rather, the bone is resorbed and the digit becomes shorter and shorter, finally disappearing.

The young man, who says he has been ill only six months, has tuberculoid (or neural) leprosy. This form of the disease often begins with an area of numbness or "pins and needles" in the skin. Later a portion of the skin may lose its color and cease to sweat or grow hair. The ability to feel a light touch (a feather or a wisp of cotton) in and around the depigmented area may be lost. Other such lesions may gradually appear and the anesthetic regions grow steadily larger.

VI

The unexpected sound of the steam calliope reverberates through the moss-hung oaks and cypress of a small peninsula not far from the point where, in Longfellow's epic poem *Evangeline*, the Acadian heroine must have slept in her boat, unaware that the fiancé she had sought for years was rowing upriver only a hundred yards away.

The sound of the calliope draws closer. Then the stern-wheeler, *Delta Queen*, all brass, teak, mahogany, and stained glass, comes around the horseshoe bend in the Mississippi on her way to New Orleans. After she disappears downriver, many of the watchers on the levee stroll across the River Road to what was formerly the Indian Camp Plantation (earlier the site of a Houma Indian village), now the National Hansen's Disease Center at Carville, Louisiana, and home to some 150 victims of leprosy from 18 countries.

One theory proposes that the Acadians, driven from Nova Scotia by the British in 1755, brought leprosy with them to Louisiana. More probably it came there with slaves from the West Indies, since there are reports of the disease in Louisiana by the mid-seventeenth century. Or perhaps it was there all the time. Whatever its origins, leprosy remains endemic in this part of Louisiana, as well as in parts of Texas, Florida, and California.

VII

Shortly after the end of World War II, I was a seaman on a navy ship bound from China to the capital of the Philippines.

Women had been cheap and plentiful in Hong Kong, and the ship's doctors and medical corpsmen were heartily sick of administering prophylaxis and treatment for venereal disease. But threats of syphilis and gonorrhea had long since lost whatever force they might once have had. So, as we neared Manila, the medical corps passed the word that most of the prostitutes of that ruined city had leprosy! We knew about leprosy, or thought we did. It made your fingers and toes fall off, maybe other things as well. My shipmates who had bragged of their sexual exploits in Hong Kong were mostly quiet when we left Manila.

VIII

The first leprosarium in Bergen was built in 1411, in the spot I described earlier. It has burned and been rebuilt several times, but St. Jørgens Hospital is still there, at 34 Kong Oscargate, only a few minutes walk from the railway station in one direction, or the center of the city in the other. In 1946, the last two patients died and it is now a leprosy museum—the only one in the world.

IX

Dr. Colin and the Superior are talking in the doctor's quarters in an African leprosarium. Dr. Colin says, "You know very well that leprophils exist. . . . Sometimes I wonder whether [Father] Damien was a leprophil. There was no need for him to become a leper in order to serve them well. A few elementary precautions—I wouldn't be a better doctor without my fingers, would I?"

"But all the same, doctor, you've said it yourself, leprosy is a psychological problem. It may be very valuable for the leper to feel loved."

"A patient can always detect whether he is loved or whether it is only his leprosy which is loved. I don't want leprosy loved. I want it eliminated."[1]

X

In the 1830s and 1840s, there was a vast increase in the number of people afflicted with leprosy in Norway. The disease was most prevalent in the western coastal districts, and particularly around Bergen. The government's response was to build a second leprosy hospital in Bergen in 1849, followed by a third eight years later. In 1856, the government began an intensive effort to register all leprosy victims in Norway. At that point there were nearly 3,000 leprosy victims in the country while, in the area around Bergen, nearly 3 of every 100 people (twenty times the country-wide incidence) had the disease.

On January 1, 1868, Gerhard Henrik Armauer Hansen, M.D., was appointed to the staff of the most recently opened leprosy hospital in Bergen. He was the eighth of fifteen children and, at twenty-seven, a powerfully built young man with powerfully held opinions. When he dutifully called on Dr. D. C. Danielssen, his chief and one of the world's most respected experts on leprosy, Armauer Hansen suddenly blurted out, "It is my conviction . . . that your opinions about leprosy are completely wrong!"[2] Hansen went on to explain that he thought leprosy was contagious, while Danielssen thought, along with most experts at the time, that it was hereditary. Danielssen had a hot temper and promptly threw the young physician out of his office. But the next day he called him back to tell him that he could have a laboratory and any equipment he needed for research on leprosy.

Armauer Hansen had always worked hard. He worked his way through medical school by tutoring younger students as much as four hours a day, and later worked as a teacher in a girl's school. He continued to work long hours after receiving his appointment in Bergen, but found time for other things as well. On January 7, 1873, he married Stephanie Danielssen, the daughter of his chief. After the honeymoon, he returned to his patients and his research.

On the last Friday in February 1873, Armauer Hansen removed nodules from each side of the nose of a nineteen-year-old leprosy victim, Johannes Giil, scraped the cut surface of the nodules, and examined the scrapings under his microscope. "Almost only round cells were seen, very few with granules of fat, some finely granulated, *others containing rod-shaped bodies which are sometimes bordered by parallel lines and sometimes pointed at both ends.* . . . Such bodies are to be found where fluid-spaces are formed by the pressure of the glass cover surrounded by a dense mass of cells. In these spaces the bodies move in the manner of 'bacteria' " (italics added). [3]

Armauer Hansen had discovered the causative agent of leprosy—but he couldn't prove it, although he had seen the small, straight rods in various preparations over the previous two years. In 1873, no one had shown a bacterium to be the cause of any human disease; this was three years before Dr. Robert Koch's discovery of the anthrax bacillus, and it would be another nine years before Koch found the tuberculosis bacterium. Criteria for establishing that a microorganism might cause an infectious disease had been laid down in 1840 by Joseph Henle and later formalized by Robert Koch. The essence of the proof was that the organism, after being routinely found in lesions of the disease, had to be grown in pure culture, free of other organisms. The pure culture then had to produce a similar disease in experimental animals, from whose lesions the organism must be recoverable.

Although he tried mightily, Armauer Hansen failed to meet any of these requirements. Yet his discovery of the causative agent was a milestone in medical microbiology. Eighty-seven years later, the leprosy bacillus was first grown in an experimental animal; and more than a century after his discovery, there are still no generally accepted reports of growing the organisms in culture.

The leprosy bacillus is now called *Mycobacterium leprae* and the disease Hansen's disease (HD) or Hanseniasis. (Hansenitis and Hansenosis have also been proposed. Since Hansenitis means an inflamed Hansen, while Hansenosis is a diseased one, these terms are no longer used). The pejorative term "leper" has been almost entirely abandoned; many people would like to see the word "leprosy" follow it into oblivion, for reasons that will become clear later on.

The disease may have originated in India, then spread to Egypt and around the Mediterranean. The earliest evidence of the disease is in mummies of the second century B.C. Roman soldiers spread it throughout Europe. The Crusades, beginning in A.D. 1096, contributed greatly to disseminating the disease, which reached its peak in most of Europe in the twelfth century. Five hundred years later, it had mostly disappeared from Europe, although it didn't reach its peak in Norway until about 1860. Today, there are an estimated 12 to 15 million sufferers from HD around the world. Less than a fourth of them are being treated. Of those under treatment, one in four already has deformed hands or feet, or both. The highest prevalence of HD is in parts of South America (Brazil has nearly 200,000 registered patients) and Africa (where there are half a million registered cases), with substantial levels in India and Indochina. India has some 3.5 million HD victims; in some villages, one person in fourteen has the disease. The People's Republic of China has some 300,000 cases under treatment. Mexico, Spain, much of the Middle East (except Egypt), and Japan still have appreciable numbers of HD victims. Australia has some 800 arrested cases.

In those areas where the prevalence of HD is high—more than one person in ten has the disease in Zaïre and in parts of India, for example—nearly everyone is exposed to *Mycobacterium leprae*. Hansen's disease is the least infectious of all transmittable diseases, and nearly everyone who is infected by the lepra bacillus throws off the infection without ever knowing that they have had it.

A fraction of the population, however, has a defective

immune response to *M. leprae*. These people develop, after an incubation period of six months to decades, the form of the disease called tuberculoid (neural) HD. In this form, the organism is confined almost entirely to the nerves and is virtually noninfectious. It is the early form of this variety of HD in which feeling is lost in various areas of the body. This leads to severe injuries and infections that cause the loss of fingers, toes, and sometimes entire limbs. It also leads to clawing of some or all of the fingers and toes, and to muscle atrophy. Wasting of the small muscles of the face renders the victim unable to close his mouth or eyes or to control the flow of tears or saliva. When the eyelids don't completely close, the exposed portions of the eyes dry out and can readily be ulcerated by dust particles that the victim cannot feel. The end result is scarring and blindness.

Still others in the exposed population fail to destroy either all the organisms (as do most people), or most of them (as in tuberculoid HD). Such people, although they may show a normal response to most other foreign substances, cannot destroy invading *M. leprae*; either the normal immune response is missing or it is somehow suppressed.

These unfortunates contract the most severe form of the disease, lepromatous HD, in which nodules appear in large numbers on the skin of the face and ears and elsewhere. Infiltration of *M. leprae* into the eyes results in blindness, and infection of the vocal cords leads first to coarsening, then loss, of the voice. The opening in the throat may become so narrow that a tiny plug of mucus could block it altogether, so the victim lives every moment in fear of suffocation. In the era before effective treatment was available, such suffocation was the third-leading cause of death at the disease center in Carville. Finally, the nerves are also attacked, and the victim of lepromatous HD suffers first the excruciating neuritis and finally the paralysis of the tuberculoid form. Victims of lepromatous HD are never spontaneously cured and, even now, must generally be treated for life.

Untreated, a fraction of tuberculoid HD victims progress to the lepromatous form (or to intermediate forms), and a still smaller fraction apparently throw off the infection.

It's ironic that, for a very long time, leprosy was thought to be highly infectious while tuberculosis was considered as solely hereditary. So victims of HD, most of whom were only slightly infectious if at all, were locked up, while tuberculars, many of whom were highly infectious, were allowed complete freedom to move through society as they pleased. Armauer Hansen's wife died of tuberculosis at twenty-seven, just ten months after they were married.

Even untreated lepromatous HD is only slightly infectious. Infection probably arises from contact with droplets containing *M. leprae* expelled when the HD victim blows his or her nose, coughs, or sneezes. The families of untreated lepromatous HD victims are obviously the ones at greatest risk of infection. Even here the incidence of secondary infection is less than 1 percent (actually 0.68 percent in one study of 22,656 contacts), despite the presence of *M. leprae* in the nasal secretions and in the breast milk of nursing mothers.[4]

The message is clear. More than ninety-nine of every hundred persons could live in intimate contact with victims of lepromatous HD for years and never contact the disease. In tuberculoid HD, the chance of secondary infection from untreated victims is almost vanishingly small.

The present treatment of newly discovered cases of Hansen's disease illustrates these facts. If the disease is in the tuberculoid (or neural) form, the victim and his family are treated as outpatients unless there are ulcers or deformities that need special medical attention, in which case the patient is hospitalized until he can be taken care of at home. Victims of tuberculoid (or advanced lepromatous) HD need special education because of the lack of feeling in their extremities and elsewhere. If they smoke, they should use a cigarette holder to avoid charring their lips or fingers. They should never drink hot liquids from a handleless cup, and their cooking utensils should have wooden handles. Their hands and feet must be inspected carefully every day for any signs of injury or irritation that, unattended, might lead to an ulcerated wound. Soft, nailless shoes like tennis shoes are the best kind of footwear for victims of tuberculoid HD if they lack feeling in their feet.

Lepromatous HD victims should be treated more vigorously because they are slightly infectious. They are ordinarily hospitalized for several weeks and their families given prophylactic treatment. Then the patient is put on an outpatient basis, returning only for periodic checkups, or for treatment of any deformities resulting from the disease.

In the United States, there are 2,000 to 3,000 HD victims, and an additional 100 to 200 new cases, mostly among immigrants, are diagnosed each year (244 in 1981). Three U.S. Public Health Service hospitals, well staffed and equipped for the treatment and rehabilitation of HD victims free of charge, were located in San Francisco; Carville, Louisiana; and Staten Island, New York. Unfortunately, the Reagan administration closed two of the three; only Carville remains. Area clinics exist, however, in Los Angeles, San Francisco, San Diego, Seattle, Staten Island, Boston, New Orleans, and Miami as of April 1982.

Among the approximately 800,000 immigrants from Scandinavia to America during the nineteenth century were several hundred HD victims; in 1888, Armauer Hansen visited the United States to check on the status of the disease here. He concluded that HD had not appeared in any of the descendants of the Norwegian leprosy victims, and he ascribed this, in part, to the fact that "Everywhere, *even among the Norwegians,* great cleanliness is observed" (italics added).[5] Armauer Hansen was not only being rather severe with his immigrant countrymen, he also missed a case of HD in an American-born descendant of Norwegian immigrants who were themselves free of the disease. Seven other such cases have been reported from Minnesota, the most recent in 1921 in a two-year-old girl.[6]

Of the 1,432 new cases of HD reported in the United States from 1967 to 1976, 344 were native-born and 87 percent of them came from six states (Louisiana, Florida, Texas, New York, California, and Hawaii). More than half the California cases were in Los Angeles County, and nearly all the New York cases occurred in New York City. (An article in the *Journal of the American Medical Association* for June 18, 1982, points out that more than 300 cases of HD are under treatment in New York City. About 60 percent are lepromatous [or borderline lepromatous], the largest ethnic group is Hispanic, and virtually all cases were imported. Only about one in six of the infected people had known prior contact with an HD victim.) In both these states, and in Florida, nearly all cases were imported. The bulk of the new cases in both Louisiana and Texas, however, were in natives of the two states. Fewer than one in five of the new Hawaiian cases were native-born, and only one fourth of those newly infected in the continental United States were aware of contact with an HD victim. In late February 1982, U.S. and Mexican health officials met to discuss an outbreak of HD in Juarez, Mexico, across the Rio Grande from El Paso. Dr. Luis Gomez had diagnosed forty new HD cases in Juarez in 1981, compared with only eighty-six new cases diagnosed in all Mexico in 1980. Most of the 408 active HD cases in Texas live close to the Mexican border.

XI

On the morning of December 1, 1894, seven HD victims arrived at Indian Camp Plantation on a coal barge from New Orleans. The once elegant mansion of crystal chandeliers and marble mantels, uninhabited for thirty years, was in ruins. The slave cabins, never elegant, were worse, and the grounds of the abandoned sugar plantation were a marshy sea of weeds. Christmas 1894 must have been a grim season for those first patients at Carville. On April 26, 1896, four nuns of the Daughters of Charity of St. Vincent de Paul arrived; the order still helps provide care for the patients.

In 1921 the federal government acquired the institution, but it remained essentially a prison surrounded by fences topped with barbed wire and patrolled by armed guards. At least there was a medical staff. During the twenty-seven years the institution had been run by the state of Louisiana, there had been a resident physician at Carville for only the final eighteen months.

Change was painfully slow. In June 1931 the American Legion took an interest in Carville and played an important role in ending the patients' isolation. In 1936 the patients got a public telephone so they could hear the voices of the family members they hadn't seen in years. In 1939 the swamps were drained, reducing the incidence of malaria. It was about time. In 1935–36, 42 percent of Carville patients had malaria in this rainiest parish of the rainiest state in the Union. And, in 1946, the state of Louisiana allowed (or more accurately ceased withholding the right of) Carville patients to vote in state and national elections. Two years later the barbed wire atop the fence was removed. Incredibly, the medieval practice of sterilizing outgoing mail survived at Carville until 1968.

Today, admission to the 100-building, 325-acre facility is voluntary. Patients go on public transportation, or in their own cars, to shop in Baton Rouge, Carville, or other nearby towns. Married couples may now live together in red brick cottages. It is a far cry from the days when male patients slipped through a hole in the fence and took a bootleg taxi to Minnie's Place on the outskirts of Baton Rouge to relieve their sexual frustrations. At that time, male and female patients were strictly segregated even if they were husband and wife.

The once decaying mansion is now the administration building of the Center. The present director is trim, handsome Dr. John Trautman, fifty-five, an Assistant Surgeon General of the U.S. Public Health Service (equivalent to a rear admiral in the navy). Dr. Trautman, a warm and friendly man, is a native of Omaha and son of a P.H.S. physician. He took his medical degree at Western Reserve University in Cleveland and spent six years at Carville as chief of the Clinical Branch before returning in 1968 as director.

The Carville bimonthly news magazine, *The Star*, has been supported by the American Legion honor society, the Forty and Eight, for many years.

The Star was founded by the incredible Stanley Stein. That wasn't his real name. When Sidney Maurice Levyson left his position as owner of a San Antonio drugstore to enter Carville on March 1, 1931, he soon met Sister Laura Stricker in the Records Room. Sister Laura asked him if he had decided on a new name. She went on to explain, "There are some stupid people in the world and you must protect your loved ones from their stupidity. Perfectly healthy children have been denied the right to attend school because some member of their family was at Carville. . . . Choose a name you will be proud of some day."[7] So Sidney Levyson became Stanley Stein —it was a name he would have good reason to be proud of— although on Carville records he was case number 746. (On June 14, 1980, Sister Laura celebrated her sixtieth anniversary as a member of the Daughters of Charity of St. Vincent de Paul. She had been at Carville for fifty-five of her sixty years in the order.)

Shortly after his arrival at Carville, Stanley Stein and a few other patients started the weekly newspaper called the *Sixty-Six Star*. As a high-school student in the Texas hill town of Boerne (the natives call it "Burney"), Stein had written a column for the Boerne *Star*. In 1931, Carville was known as U.S. Marine Hospital No. 66, hence the paper's name. In Stein's hands, *The Star* became a potent weapon for changing many of the terrible aspects of the patients' lives at Carville. In a series of articles he campaigned for new projection equipment and better movies, for a better infirmary, a new recreation hall, better contact with the outside world, and for abolition of the term "leper." In addition to all this he wrote an advice to the lovelorn column for *The Star*, organized a little theater group, and began a series of other events that made the patients of Carville into a community instead of a group of isolated and lonely people.

Stein's lepromatous HD got steadily worse. He began to lose feeling in his hands. More lesions appeared on his face and he lost the sight of his left eye. He developed inflammation in his right eye (iritis) and applied hot packs to ease the agonizing pain. But, lacking feeling, he often scalded his hands while trying to treat his eyes. At thirty-eight, six years after he entered Carville, Stanley Stein was totally blind. All his life he had been an omnivorous reader, but with no feeling in his fingers he couldn't even learn Braille. Stein was devastated by the loss of sight and he withdrew from all the activities he had begun. But not for long.

Soon he was back doing what he did best—fighting. Stein campaigned vigorously for a new post office, for removal of the barbed wire from the top of the cyclone fence, for restoration of the patients' right to vote, for weekend passes, and for anything else he thought would make Carville a more pleasant place. And he got results. He became a friend of actress Tallulah Bankhead and columnist Bob Considine. In 1961, on *The Star*'s thirtieth anniversary, President John F. Kennedy praised the paper and its indomitable editor "for immeasurably adding to the world's understanding of Hansen's disease."

Early that same year Stanley Stein broke his arm. Two days later he broke his hip. His hearing gradually failed. Just before Christmas 1967 he died. The news magazine he founded now has a circulation of about 80,000 in all 50 states and 118 foreign countries. Stein wrote in his autobiography: "I certainly wanted *The Star* to be a friend to the friendless, but I dared not hope then that it could ever become the voice of the voiceless, a cry of despair from those without the camp,* an appeal for justice."[8] *The Star* became all that, and more.

* From the injunction in Leviticus that lepers must live without (outside of) the tribal camp.

President Reagan sent the paper a congratulatory letter in October 1981, when *The Star* celebrated its fortieth anniversary. The present editor is Louis Boudreaux, also blinded by the disease, who entered Carville just three years after Stanley Stein.

Hansen's disease was treated for centuries with a variety of potions, including the painful injection of chaulmoogra oil, that were of little or no use. Then, in March 1941, Dr. Guy Paget and his associates at Carville first tried a complex derivative of dapsone (an inexpensive drug closely related to the sulfonamides). To their delight, it worked. Of twenty-two victims of advanced lepromatous HD, twenty-one clearly benefited from the treatment. The twenty-second was Stanley Stein.

The complex derivative of dapsone only worked because it was broken down in the body to dapsone, so the simpler and less expensive dapsone could be used just as well. In tuberculoid HD, treatment with dapsone tablets can be stopped after five years so long as the patient is watched carefully for signs of relapse. This drug, in the concentrations usually used, does not kill *M. leprae* but prevents it from growing. Intramuscular injection of another dapsone derivative (acedapsone) maintains a high level of the drug in the blood for more than two months. This is useful for treating contacts of HD victims, but its use in lepromatous cases may lead to dapsone resistance.

As expected, dapsone-resistant *M. leprae* began to appear. Of Dr. Paget's original twenty-two patients, half were infected by dapsone-resistant *M. leprae* by the 1950s. Dapsone resistance appears in lepromatous patients who have been treated for years with the drug. Then their disease begins to progress despite dapsone treatment. Since treatment of the lepromatous form is lifelong, and many sufferers are diagnosed as children, this is obviously a serious matter. But resistance was ultimately found in newly diagnosed cases as well. These victims had the misfortune to be infected from the beginning by a dapsone-resistant strain of the organism. Unfortunately, dapsone resistance is genetically stable, hence the resistant organisms don't revert to dapsone sensitivity with the passage of time. This so-called primary resistance is an increasingly serious problem. Currently, four of every ten newly diagnosed cases in the African republic of Mali, for example, have primary dapsone resistance.[9] The current strategy is to treat all new cases of HD with combinations of drugs if the victims have a high level of *M. leprae* in their tissues.

Another problem with the treatment (besides occasionally fatal reactions to the drugs) is that, even after ten years of dapsone therapy (or two years of therapy with more potent drugs that kill more than 99 percent of the *M. leprae* after a single dose), viable, drug-sensitive *M. leprae* can be recovered from patients. These persisters, as the organisms are called, are metabolically inactive and do not multiply. Presumably it is the persisters that are responsible for relapse many years, or even decades, after treatment has ended.

It is extremely difficult to study an infectious disease unless it—or something close to it and caused by the same organism—can be produced in an experimental animal. Then the progress of the infection can be studied and various modes of therapy tried before they are applied to human cases. When dapsone was first available, the only experimental animals available were the human victims of HD. Nothing was known about the drug's efficacy against the disease, the most effective dose rate, or possible serious side effects. Because of the lack of an animal model, this essential information was obtained from studies on humans. In the early years of dapsone use, the practice was to increase the dose slowly over a long period of time to avoid unpleasant (and occasionally fatal) reactions to the drug. This practice, now largely abandoned, was a major factor in selecting drug-resistant *M. leprae* in human patients, since only those few organisms genetically equipped to grow in the presence of a low concentration of the drug could survive and multiply. Had an animal model been available in the 1940s, this tragic result might have been avoided.

It was known that *M. leprae* grew best at temperatures

below those of most animals. That is why its manifestations in humans appear mostly in cooler areas such as the skin or the superficial nerves. In 1960, Charles Shepard, M.D., at what was then called the U.S.P.H.S. Communicable Disease Center in Atlanta (since 1980 known as the Centers for Disease Control), had a brilliant idea. The footpads of rodents and other animals are at a lower temperature than the rest of the body. Would the HD bacillus grow in mouse footpads, for example? Dr. Shepard injected the footpads of mice with *M. leprae* from a human victim and waited. He waited a long time. The HD bacillus doubles its numbers in the footpad in eleven to thirteen days (most bacteria have doubling times in favorable circumstances of from twenty minutes to a day). If Dr. Shepard attempted to speed things up by injecting large numbers of *M. leprae* at one time, this stimulated the mouse's immune system and the infection was promptly wiped out. It was months before Charles Shepard could be sure that *M. leprae* was growing in the mouse footpad.

As with most animal models, Dr. Shepard had produced an artificial disease. Normal mice are resistant to HD and eventually destroy the infection. The disease does not spread in the mouse as it does in humans and so does not produce similar manifestations. But Shepard's discovery was the most important advance in HD research since the discovery of the organism because, for the first time, it provided a relatively pure population of *M. leprae* for study that was far more convenient than taking material from a human victim of the disease. It also offered a system, albeit an agonizingly slow one, for testing drugs and potential vaccines for their ability to suppress the infection in an animal.

The third giant step in HD research began on Tuesday, February 10, 1970, when Waldemar F. Kirchheimer, M.D., Ph.D., chief of the Laboratory Research Branch at the Carville Center, and Eleanor E. Storrs, Ph.D., of the Gulf South Research Institute in New Iberia, Louisiana, inoculated *M. leprae* from a human case into the skin of the ears and abdomens of four nine-banded armadillos. As in all phases of HD research and treatment, great patience was required. But, sixteen months later, on May 24, 1971, Kirchheimer and Storrs agreed that lesions were visible at the sites of inoculation in one of the male armadillos, although in none of the other inoculated animals. These lesions contained large numbers of M. *leprae* and, most important of all, the organisms were also found in normal skin remote from the inoculation site.

Further painstaking work showed that, two or three years after inoculation, a large proportion of armadillos injected with M. *leprae* had a disseminated form of HD in which the organisms were found in vast quantities in the animals' spleens and livers. One armadillo could yield up to 10 trillion (10 million millions) M. *leprae*.

Armadillos are primitive creatures related to anteaters and sloths. Native to Mexico and South America, the nine-banded armadillo arrived in the southern United States some 150 years ago and spread east from Texas to Florida, and north into Oklahoma, Arkansas, and Georgia. They now number some 10 million in the United States, although the number in captivity is only a few hundred. As a source of M. *leprae* for study and for vaccine production, armadillos are superb. They have a body temperature of 90–92° F (32–5° C), and a lifespan of a dozen years or more. But they have one major drawback. They resolutely refuse to breed in captivity, so the supply of armadillos for laboratory studies must be constantly replenished by trapping the wild animals. This presents both a small problem and a large mystery.

About 10 percent of the armadillos trapped in southern Louisiana already have HD. Using wild animals for research purposes is a problem because the genetic makeup of the animals is obviously uncontrolled and there is no way to tell to what diseases the animals have been exposed. It is especially aggravating when the animals already have the disease with which you wanted to inoculate them, since you can't tell how long they've had it or with what strain they were infected.

The mystery is: How do armadillos contract HD in the wild? For a clue, we return to Norway to Lorentz M. Irgens, M.D., of the Institute for Hygiene and Social Medicine, of the University of Bergen. Dr. Irgens was intrigued by the historically high concentration of Norwegian HD victims (over 8,000 registered after 1856) in the area around Bergen. His investigations revealed that the district with the highest incidence of HD in the nineteenth century was the one with the highest average summertime humidity, Naustdal. When samples of sphagnum mosses were collected from the Naustdal health district, nearly a third of them harbored organisms resembling mycobacteria in their unique staining properties. Some of these organisms were apparently able to grow in mouse footpads. Although these studies are incomplete, they suggest that *M. leprae* may have an ecological niche from which both humans and animals may be infected. Whether this is true remains to be seen. The crucial point is whether the moss organisms are really *M. leprae*.

It was long suspected either that the infected wild armadillos had escaped from the Gulf South Research Institute or that wild armadillos had been infected by eating the incompletely incinerated remains of an experimentally infected animal. Armadillos are known to be cannibalistic and the bodies of animals dead of the disease contain enormous levels of *M. leprae*. Moreover, all infected animals were trapped in an area contiguous with the Research Institute although as much as thirty-nine miles away.

Recently, however, an infected armadillo has been trapped on the other side of the Atchafalaya and Mississippi rivers. Although the heavily armored armadillos can hold their breath for several minutes and commonly cross small streams by walking across the bottom, they're unlikely to cross rivers as vast as the Mississippi this way. So the wild armadillos in southern Louisiana are probably naturally infected in some way.

The infection of wild armadillos with *M. leprae* is not a

serious detriment to the use of this animal as a research tool since there is no lack of HD-free armadillos in other parts of Louisiana and elsewhere in the South. More recent work has suggested that the European hedgehog, athymic mice (and possibly athymic rats),* all of which breed well in captivity, offer additional models for HD research. A recent exciting finding is the existence in, and transmission of HD from, a particular kind of monkey (the sooty mangabey) in which the disease closely resembles that in humans.[10]

The problems involved in the worldwide control of HD are staggering. Of the estimated 12 to 15 million cases, only about one fourth are registered by the health authorities of their home countries and are thus potentially available for treatment. But even after they are registered, what then?

An encouraging note comes from an experiment in HD control being carried out on the Mediterranean island of Malta, under the direction of Prof. Dr. Enno Freerksen of the Institute for Experimental Biology and Medicine in Borstal, West Germany. On Malta, all known HD victims have been treated with the mixture of the antileprotics prothionamide and dapsone known as Isoprodian, and the anti-TB drug isoniazid, to eradicate both tuberculosis and HD in a single course of treatment. The combination of two antileprotics virtually eliminates resistance problems. Treatment may be supplemented with daily administration of rifampin, a semi-synthetic antibiotic that kills 99 percent of $M.$ $leprae$ in a single dose. Two hundred fifty patients are involved in the study. Each of them was examined both clinically and micro-biologically once a month to follow changes in their physical condition and the disappearance of living $M.$ $leprae$ from their tissues. Some patients required treatment for only six months, others for three times as long. All patients completed treatment at least seven years ago and, according to the most recent report, there have been no relapses among the HD victims.[11]

---

* Animals genetically lacking a thymus gland or from which the gland is removed at birth and which are thus immuno-deficient.

If this surprising finding continues to hold up, it means that HD may be eradicated by comparatively brief treatment. A larger scale application of the same method is now going on among Paraguay's more than 5,000 HD victims, and in India and Africa. Other work in Malaysia suggests that, following intensive short-term therapy, the relapse rate of HD victims is about 1 percent a year. The authors of a recent paper in *The Lancet* (May 29, 1982) report that rifampicin once a month plus daily dapsone gives results as good as those obtained when both drugs are given each day, but at a cost of only one tenth as much.

Unfortunately, rifampin is not approved by the FDA for the general treatment of HD in the United States, it renders birth control pills ineffective (in the United States alone there are more than 300 women of child-bearing age with HD), it has some undesirable side effects, and it is very expensive. A year's supply for a single HD patient costs $300 or more, while the average annual income in India, for example, is less than half that. Dapsone, by contrast, costs only a few dollars a year. A current plan to combat the increasing problem of dapsone-resistant *M. leprae* is to give rifampin (plus dapsone and another antileprotic-clofazimine) once a month at a yearly cost of approximately $50.

All drugs used in the treatment of HD produce various HD reactions. These result from a sudden stimulation of the body's defenses against the lepra bacillus, and occur in untreated patients as well, although not so frequently. These reactions—which, not surprisingly, are much more severe in the lepromatous form of the disease—may cause severe pain in the nerves, joints, and bones, and if not adequately treated may lead to serious and irreversible damage to the patient. The serious reactions of lepromatous patients are most effectively treated with thalidomide, oddly enough, and with steroids. But patients living in isolated areas may quite reasonably associate taking their daily ration of dapsone tablets with the thoroughly unpleasant reactions and stop taking the pills until they feel better. Intermittent administration of the drug is a strong contributor to the spreading development of dapsone resistance.

The World Health Organization (WHO) has a Therapy of Leprosy project (THELEP), the goal of which is to develop better drugs and treatment regimes for HD. In 1974, WHO also began an IMMLEP project to study the immunology of leprosy, with the goal of producing a vaccine against the disease by 1984. The WHO experts agreed that this was essential because of the problems of drug resistance and the persistence of M. *leprae* even after years of drug therapy.

WHO recently announced that trials of a new HD vaccine made from the livers and spleens of HD-infected armadillos would be conducted in the first nine months of 1982. The trial will be carried out in the United States, the United Kingdom, and Scandinavia to avoid charges that drug testing is being done on unsuspecting Third World country inhabitants, even though Third World inhabitants will be the principal beneficiaries of a successful trial.

The potential efficacy of vaccination against HD is controversial. If there is no host for the disease but man, as is probably the case for smallpox, then, as with smallpox, an intensive vaccination program might eradicate it.

A vaccine seeks to mimic natural infection by stimulating the body to produce antibodies to substances (antigens) present on the surface of the killed or weakened virus or bacteria in the vaccine. Thus, when a natural infection with the same organism occurs, the body's immune system has already stockpiled the weapons needed to destroy the infecting agent. The basic assumption is that the body responds to the vaccine by producing either antibodies that label the invading organisms as foreign, and thus lead to their destruction, or specific cell types (lymphocytes and macrophages) that cooperatively recognize and destroy the infecting organism. These two different types of response are referred to as humoral (antibody) or cellular (lymphocyte and macrophage) immunity. Humoral immunity seems to play no significant part in the body's response against M. *leprae*. Although antibodies to the organism are made, they don't clear up the infection. The cellular immune response in HD victims fails as well— partially in the case of the tuberculoid form, totally in the lepromatous form. This failure may have a genetic component.

Unfortunately, in much of the world, half or more of the cases of HD are the lepromatous form. If the victim of lepromatous HD does not mount an effective immune response to the billions of M. *leprae* in his or her body, why should the injection of a few million killed or weakened lepra bacilli alter that tragic fact? As Dr. Kirchheimer of Carville puts it: "I maintain, as I always have, that those people who happen to be highly susceptible to HD will not and cannot benefit from vaccination. . . . Those individuals [with lepromatous HD] cannot become immune because of a defect in their immune systems. . . . Obviously, the WHO Immunology of Leprosy Project Group does not share this view."[12] The present plan is to grow the organisms in armadillos in Louisiana, ship the tissues to Mill Hill, England, for purification of the bacteria, then send the bacteria to investigators in the United States and Norway for further testing.[13]

If and when a vaccine is available, who is to be vaccinated? Even in a region of severely endemic HD, 90 percent or more of the population, although exposed to the lepra bacillus, are able to throw off the infection. A few percent of the inhabitants have a weak cellular immunity (and are thus at risk of contracting the tuberculoid form). They might be helped by vaccination to respond more effectively. Those potentially susceptible to lepromatous HD probably will not respond at all. This means that 100 percent of the population must be vaccinated for the 2 to 3 percent (or less) that may benefit. Side effects from any mass vaccination are a certainty, and the relatively high risk-benefit ratio makes widespread vaccination against HD seem dubious at this point.

There is no vaccine currently in hand, however, and evaluation of the field trials set to begin in 1982 may take a decade. Then the picture may be clearer and perhaps more encouraging. After all, nearly 200 years passed between the development of an effective smallpox vaccine and the apparent worldwide eradication of the disease. It is certain that the debate over the utility of an HD vaccine has stimulated fundamental research into HD immunology that will extend our knowledge of the immune response in many ways.

Production of adequate amounts of the vaccine at a reasonable cost is another hurdle to be cleared. At the moment, M. leprae can only be grown in large quantities in armadillos. It's reasonable (though it may be wrong) to assume that each armadillo three years after infection will yield some 4,000 doses of vaccine. To protect the 2 billion (2,000 million) people who may be at risk of contracting HD, about half a million armadillos will be needed. The total number in captivity is under 500. Although there are an estimated 10 million armadillos in the American South, the cost of the facilities for housing, feeding, and caring for half a million armadillos—which weigh up to 11 pounds apiece—is staggering, especially in the present era when funds for public health efforts are being severely cut or altogether obliterated.

In the July 1982 issue of *Infection and Immunity* there appeared a report of the preparation of monoclonal antibodies* to M. leprae. This immunological approach would, in

---

* The newly developed monoclonal antibody technique is one of the most exciting aspects of biotechnology. It involves immunizing a mouse with an antigen (in this case, fragments of M. leprae) so that the mouse's spleen cells (lymphocytes) will manufacture cells that make antibody specifically against each of the various antigens in the mixture (or against various portions of a single antigen). The lymphocytes, which are short-lived in culture, are then fused with tumor cells, which will grow indefinitely in culture, and clones (descendants of a single cell) are selected that make only a single antibody rather than the complex mixture made by the entire spleen. The result is antibody of a specificity heretofore undreamed of.

principle, make it possible to detect antibodies to M. *leprae* in the blood serum of individuals during the long interval (the incubation period) before clinical symptoms appeared. Timely treatment of such individuals might abort the infection.

Robert C. Hastings, M.D., Ph.D., chief of the Pharmacological Research Department at the Carville Center, and the current editor of the *International Journal of Leprosy*, estimates the cost of obtaining vaccine from a single armadillo at $2,500 (food, housing, and vaccine production).[14] Calculation of the cost of obtaining vaccine from half a million armadillos is left as an exercise for the reader.

Meanwhile, HD victims the world over continue to suffer the legacy of fear and loathing that was given early expression in the Old Testament (which carried it over from Assyro-Babylonic practice), and continued in the New Testament and in the Koran:

> When a man shall have in the skin of his flesh a rising, a scab, or bright spot, and it be in the skin of his flesh like the plague of leprosy, then he shall be brought unto . . . the priest . . . and the priest shall look on him, and pronounce him unclean. . . . He is a leprous man, he is unclean. . . . And the leper in whom the plague is, his clothes shall be rent, and his head bare, and he shall put a covering upon his upper lip, and shall cry, Unclean, unclean. All the days wherein the plague shall be in him he shall be defiled; he is unclean: he shall dwell alone; without the camp shall his habitation be.[15]

About the time this vicious bit of folklore was being received by Moses and his band of primitive nomads, the same barbaric philosophy was being acted on by Ramses II, pharaoh of the urbane and cultivated Egyptians, who ordered 80,000 lepers confined in a settlement on the edge of the Sahara. The tragedy of such injunctions was that leprosy is one of the great imitators in medicine. So the victims of any sort of skin disorder—acne, scabies, eczema, fungal infections, scurvy, impetigo, psoriasis, syphilis, skin cancer, boils, ringworm, seborrhea, and many others—were equally at risk of lifetime banishment and persecution.

It would be pleasing to report that such attitudes no longer exist. Unfortunately, they do. They are even official government policy in some quite highly developed countries. Dr. Robert Gelbar, formerly of the P.H.S. Hospital in San Francisco, tells of a young man who promptly committed suicide on learning that he had HD, despite the fact that every effort was made to persuade him that the diagnosis would have very little effect on his future life. Among Dr. Gelbar's patients there are husbands who have been treated for years but have never told their wives of their disease, and vice versa.

Lynda Zaunbrecher, M.D., of the Carville medical staff, tells the following story:

> I was on a bus on my way to Carville. The man sitting next to me started to talk to me and asked me where I was going. He seemed surprised that there was a P.H.S. hospital at Carville. I explained that it was a speciality hospital, and that its speciality is Hansen's disease (HD). His next question was "What is HD?" I went on to explain that it is a skin disease that produces skin lesions that sometimes become anesthetic and if un-checked, can destroy peripheral nerves and also affect the eyes, ears, and nose. Trauma due to lack of sensation often causes injury to hands and feet. I also mentioned that it is only slightly contagious. He then asked, "Aren't you afraid of catching it?" I explained how extremely small the risk is, and how with modern drug therapy, a patient could rapidly become non-contagious. He said he was surprised that he'd never heard of the disease before. I said, "You probably have, it's also

known as leprosy." From that moment on, his manner totally changed. He inched over to the edge of his seat and looked around the bus (probably to find another seat, but the bus was full). He said that he couldn't believe I was actually going to go there. The point of the story is that the facts about HD did not frighten him very much. It was the word "leprosy" that did. He wasn't petrified by the disease itself, only its name.[16]

No wonder, then, that *The Star* opposes use of the word "leprosy"—it still inspires fear and loathing around the world.

An Israeli psychologist, Dr. Liora Meisels, interviewed many of Israel's 300 HD patients. One of the interviews took place by flashlight in a car parked in a public parking lot; another when none of a patient's family was home. Even the patient's wife did not know he had the disease. After patients were no longer infectious, they continued to regard themselves as such, keeping special teacups for guests, for example, so that they would not have to use those the patient might have used. They suffered, in Dr. Meisels's phrase, from "the stigma of the stigma," seeing it as much more severe than even an intolerant society perceived it to be.[17]

NBC Evening News, on May 27, 1974, presented the story of the adoption by Janet and Louis Marchese of two girls from the leprosy village of St. Lazarus in Suwon, South Korea. Korea has some 80,000 victims of HD and an official attitude toward them that Moses would wholly approve. Completely healthy relatives of such victims cannot find jobs, adequate housing, or even attend school with the children of other families. The Korean word for the children of HD victims is *mi-kama*; it means, "Not yet infected." The implication of inexorable infection is, as we have seen, palpable nonsense. St. Lazarus village is on a remote mountainside, and children born there must live, work, and marry within the village.

The Cho family of St. Lazarus decided to give up their

two daughters for adoption in the United States so that the children would have the chance for a decent life. Louis Marchese, a mustachioed, husky policeman in Mahopec, New York, and his voluble, dark-haired wife, Janet, already had two children, but they agreed to adopt the Chos' daughters. In all, eight children from five families were adopted by American couples. It took four years and four separate acts of Congress for this to be achieved.[18] It is also interesting that, since the Vanderbilt University Television News Archives were established in August 1968, the only recorded mention of HD on television evening news has been in connection with the five Korean children. The fact that there are several thousand HD victims in America has never been mentioned.

There are hopeful signs that, although the total number of Hansen's disease victims in the world has not changed appreciably for many years, new approaches to drug therapy and the possible development of an effective vaccine may make control of the disease a reality throughout much of the world in the next few decades.

The other battle to be waged is against ignorance, superstition, and fear. This battle may be much harder than that against the disease itself. Here, at least, is a battle in which we can all take part by spreading the truth about HD to anyone willing to listen.

The Great Bicentennial Swine Flu Caper

In the first wintry weeks of the Bicentennial Year, an imaginative young soldier marching at night on frozen ground might have felt some kinship with the ragged soldiers of the Continental Army slogging with rag-wrapped feet through the snow of Valley Forge, or rowing with numbed fingers across the icy Delaware River as General Washington made his daring Christmas Day raid on the Hessian encampment at Trenton, New Jersey. But, although the point where George Washington stepped ashore that famous night was only a brisk day's march away, Private David Lewis, nineteen, a new recruit from Ashley Falls, Massachusetts, had more pressing things on his mind. He was very ill. He should not have joined the forced march in the bitter cold. Now he knew that he must drop out.

The day before, Tuesday, February 3, 1976, he had visited the outpatient clinic of Fort Dix complaining of a cold. He had a moderate temperature (100.4°F), and the medic who examined him did not consider him ill enough to hospitalize. Instead, he was told to stay in his company's barracks for forty-eight hours and then report to the outpatient clinic before returning to duty.

Private Lewis had arrived at Fort Dix, New Jersey, a month earlier for seven weeks of Basic Combat Training. By now he had good friends among the 200 other fledgling soldiers of Company E-1, and he hadn't wanted to chicken out of the training march on Wednesday night because of a cold.

But he was feverish and nauseated. His head and body ached, and his throat was dry and sore. His strength failed rapidly. Even with frequent rests, he dropped farther and farther behind the column. Then, only a quarter mile from the end of the march, he collapsed and was taken to the emergency room in an ambulance. By the time the ambulance climbed the slippery hill and slid to a stop outside the emergency room entrance behind Walson Army Hospital, Private David Lewis was dead.

Thus began the incredible story of what has been termed, even in circumspect medical journals, a fiasco and a debacle—the great Bicentennial swine flu caper of 1976.

That year was the two hundredth anniversary of the Declaration of Independence; it was an election year, and it was also the year that swine influenza reemerged as a transmissible human disease after nearly fifty years of relative obscurity.

It is not unheard of for young soldiers to die during strenuous physical activity—the commonest cause is undetected heart disease—but neither was it a matter taken lightly by the Fort Dix medical officers. An autopsy was performed to determine the cause of Private Lewis's death. The pathologist did not have far to seek once he opened the young soldier's chest. David Lewis's right lung was dark red and grotesquely swollen with blood and fluid that welled out under the scalpel blade. His left lung was smaller but similar in appearance. It was a typical case of fatal viral pneumonia, a rare complication of influenza.

David Lewis had arrived at Fort Dix on January 6 as the camp repopulated after the Christmas holidays. During most of that month the effective temperature at the base (taking into account the wind chill factor) was only rarely as high as 0°F. It sank as low as −43°, and was −10°F for two bone-chilling weeks. David Lewis's was certainly not the first case of flu at Fort Dix in that intensely cold winter of 1976. Some incoming soldiers and recruits had brought influenza to the camp with them and it had spread rapidly. Among the approximately 6,000 recruits, over 400 had been hospitalized with acute respiratory disease by the end of January. For every case serious enough to be hospitalized, there were many more victims who were told to stay in bed, or at least inside, for a couple of days. David Lewis was not hospitalized. Ironically, by the time of his death on February 4, the Fort Dix influenza epidemic had already peaked, although the number of weekly admissions to the hospital for acute respiratory disease did not drop below 100 until mid-April.

Martin Goldfield, M.D., was head of the Division of Laboratories and Epidemiology of the New Jersey Department of Health. Samples of mucus and tissues from David Lewis's throat and lungs eventually arrived in his Trenton laboratory by courier, along with other samples from both civilian and military patients in New Jersey. Antimicrobials (antibiotics) were added to the samples to prevent bacterial growth, and portions of them were put in vessels containing monkey cell cultures, while other portions were injected into fertilized chicken eggs containing embryos nine to eleven days old. Both these procedures were designed to give any viruses present in the samples a medium in which they could multiply rapidly. The monkey cell cultures were incubated at human body temperature for a week; the fertile eggs were ready for viral harvest in two or three days.

There are three classes of influenza viruses named, in the order of their discovery, A, B, and C. Type C flu virus is common but not dangerous; it causes an illness resembling the common cold. Type B is common enough and sometimes dangerous, but it is genetically more stable than type A and has never caused worldwide epidemics, or pandemics as they are called. Type A flu viruses, on the other hand, are both common and unstable; they were responsible for the Asian flu pandemic of 1957–58 and the Hong Kong pandemic of 1968–69.

Dr. Goldfield's technicians sought to answer three questions about the samples coming into the Trenton laboratory. First, did they contain viruses and, if so, how many and what kind? Public health laboratories around the world constantly watch for the emergence of new variants of influenza virus because such variants, to which most of the population has no immunity, have the potential for causing widespread illness. Dr. Goldfield's technicians were the first to discover that something strange was going on at Fort Dix.

It was easy to tell which samples contained viruses. A technician carefully added a known volume of the diluted samples to shallow wells in a clear plastic plate. Other wells were filled with the same sample at progressively higher dilutions. A suspension of chicken red blood cells was then added to all the wells, the mixture was gently stirred, and left at room temperature for half an hour or more.

In those wells containing no virus, the blood cells settled to the bottom in a compact red button. Where viruses were present, the compact button of red cells was absent; instead, the bottom of the well was covered by a thin film. This is because many viruses have the ability to cause red blood cells to agglutinate, or clump together. The virus particle binds to a pair of red cells. If enough virus is present, these same red cells may bind another virus particle, and then another, until all the red cells are linked together by virus particles in a diffuse mat that settles toward the bottom of the well. This is called the hemagglutination test.

When the laboratory technician returned to inspect the

plates, she found some rows of wells that contained only the compact red button of blood cells at the bottom, indicating the absence of agglutinating viruses. Other rows showed a diffuse film of agglutinated red cells in the wells containing a high concentration of the sample. The remaining wells in that row contained compacted red cells, since the concentration of virus particles was too low to cause red cell agglutination. The technician could estimate the number of viral particles (the titer) in the original sample by taking the dilution factor into account. The higher the titer, the higher the dilution of the sample that still caused the red cells to agglutinate, and the farther across the row of wells the diffuse mats of red cells extended.

The questions of which samples contained virus and how much were answered. The next question was: What kind of viruses were they? Dr. Goldfield's technicians were unable to answer this question.

Humans and other animals respond to influenza infection by making antibodies to the influenza virus.* Antibodies to influenza A virus do not react with influenza B virus. Moreover, antibodies to variants of A virus bind strongly only to that variant and weakly, if at all, to other variants. Antibody preparations specific for the common varieties of flu viruses are stockpiled in public health laboratories. It's a simple matter for an experienced technician to classify a flu virus by testing it against a variety of influenza virus antibodies and noting which antibodies inhibit the hemagglutination reaction.

A batch of throat samples from Fort Dix had arrived in the Trenton laboratory on the evening of January 29, even before Private Lewis's last march. A second batch arrived late the next day. Six of the first eight samples from Fort Dix

---

* Antibodies are large protein molecules that combine in a highly specific way with foreign substances, or antigens, thus neutralizing their effects.

contained flu viruses. Four of those six were clearly influenza A/Victoria, one of the flu strains afflicting humanity around the world in the fall and winter of 1975–76.

It was the other two samples that were baffling. Although they seemed to be typical influenza viruses, they did not react with the antibodies to either influenza A or B that were available in the New Jersey laboratory. The tests were repeated, with the same results.

Only half-convinced of the validity of the data, but not wanting to miss a potentially important observation, Martin Goldfield telephoned Dr. Walter Dowdle of the World Health Organization (WHO) Influenza Center for the Americas at the federal Center for Disease Control (CDC) in Atlanta, Georgia. Dr. Goldfield said that, although he suspected the findings were not significant, he would ship some samples harvested from eggs newly infected with the two mystery virus samples to Dr. Dowdle by plane.

By then a second batch of eleven samples from Fort Dix was ready for assay. Four of them contained influenza virus, three of which were A/Victoria. The remaining sample behaved like the two mystery virus samples in the first group. A fourth sample of the unusual virus or viruses turned up in a later batch. A week later, swabs from David Lewis's throat yielded the fifth and last sample of the unidentified virus(es).

Meanwhile Dr. Dowdle and his staff in Atlanta were at work trying to identify the viruses that had arrived from Trenton. Flu viruses are named according to their type, the place in which they were discovered, and the year. The A/Victoria samples from New Jersey were quickly identified by Dr. Dowdle's staff as A/Victoria/75, but the mystery viruses were neither A/Victoria/75 nor B/Hong Kong/72, the two influenza viruses then most widely distributed around the world.

Additional material was needed for further testing. The hemagglutination test alone requires about 10 million virus particles; the unknown virus samples were therefore inoculated into fertilized eggs on the day of their arrival in Atlanta so that the virus could multiply. On Saturday, February 7, the fluids from the inoculated eggs were checked, but gave only weak activity and were reinoculated into embryonated eggs.

On Thursday, February 12, Dr. Dowdle and his assistants made a startling discovery. All five samples of the unknown virus(es) from Fort Dix had their ability to agglutinate red blood cells inhibited by antibody to the influenza virus isolated from North American swine in both 1975 and 1976. The swine virus had two slightly different subpopulations. So did the virus from Fort Dix. This strongly suggested that the original source of the Fort Dix infections was a pig suffering from the porcine form of influenza and that only a single virus was involved; all five samples were the same. Although swine influenza virus had been isolated before in recent years from humans in contact with pigs, it had never been involved in human-to-human transmission, yet that was what had surely happened at Fort Dix.

When they studied the Fort Dix virus in the electron microscope, the CDC scientists saw roughly spherical virus particles whose outer surfaces were covered with spikes or rods. These projections were of two types. One was a molecule involved in binding the viral particles to animal cells. Since it is this reaction that causes red cells to agglutinate, this large protein molecule is called hemagglutinin. It is also antigenic— that is, it stimulates the production of antibody molecules designed to bind specifically to it. There are three variants of the hemagglutinin (H) antigen found on human influenza viruses; on the swine flu virus, the hemagglutinin molecule was designated H_{1sw}.

The second type of projection from the surface of the virus was another protein, an enzyme called neuraminidase. There are two variants of neuraminidase (N) antigen found on human influenza viruses, N_1 and N_2.

The virus particles were concentrated by centrifugation in Dr. Dowdle's Atlanta laboratory and their neuraminidase activity checked. In all samples of the mystery virus, the

enzyme was inhibited only by antibodies to the N_1 neuraminidase of the swine flu virus.

That same second week in February additional tests were
carried out in the Trenton laboratories. It soon became clear
that a radically new strain of influenza was abroad at Fort Dix.
It had the ability to spread person to person and it was
capable of producing fatal viral pneumonia. On Friday the
13th, Walter Dowdle and his colleagues identified the mystery
virus as one that closely resembled a swine flu virus. The Fort
Dix virus would henceforth be designated A/New Jersey/76
($H_{1sw}N_1$).

There was still one more confirmatory test: serum taken
from influenza victims a few weeks after their illness contains antibodies they have produced to whatever variety of
influenza virus has infected them. Serum from two of the
four patients from whom the swine flu virus had first been
isolated at Fort Dix was checked for the presence of antibodies
to reference strains of the swine virus. The serum from patients
with A/Victoria/75 influenza was also checked at Trenton, at
the army's Walter Reed Institute for Medical Research, and
at the CDC, Atlanta. All the laboratory results agreed. Patients
from whom swine flu virus had been isolated had serum antibodies only to swine flu and not to A/Victoria/75. Conversely,
patients from whom A/Victoria/75 had been isolated had
antibodies only to that virus and not to swine influenza. Swine
flu virus was isolated from only five patients at Fort Dix.
Ironically, David Lewis was the last. All subsequent influenza
cases at Fort Dix were A/Victoria/75. Later, more detailed
serological investigation revealed that there had been at least
230 cases of swine flu at Fort Dix between January 19 and
February 2, mostly in three companies of recruits that had 40
to 45 percent infection rates. The disease was probably transmitted in the reception center, where all the recruits had
spent their first three days. Of these several hundred cases of
swine flu, only twelve had required hospitalization. Private
Lewis was the only fatality.

The virus that killed David Lewis was unequivocally A/New Jersey/76 ($H_{1sw}N_1$); but to the news media, when the story broke, it was swine flu from beginning to end, to the great distress of the pig farmers and the meat-packing industry.

Identification of the virus that killed David Lewis brought chills to the spines of some influenza experts. It was a swine influenza virus that probably caused the greatest flu pandemic of modern times—the 1918–19 onslaught that struck 1 of every 4 Americans, killing 548,000 persons in the United States alone, and at least 20 million more in the rest of the world. That pandemic killed more people in a few months than had died in all four years of World War I. The 1918–19 pandemic was also unique in causing a very high proportion of total deaths among those twenty to forty years of age, whereas the usual fatalities from influenza occur in the very young and in the elderly, or in those at high risk because of other ailments (heart, respiratory, and kidney diseases, diabetes, and so on). Did the appearance of swine flu at Fort Dix presage another epidemic on the scale of 1918? And if so, what then?

A human influenza virus was first isolated in 1933 by a trio of scientists at the National Institute for Medical Research in London. Dr. Richard E. Shope of the Rockefeller Institute of Comparative Pathology in Princeton, New Jersey, had isolated the swine influenza virus from pigs for the first time only three years before. The human flu virus isolated in London in 1933 closely resembled the virus isolated from swine by Shope. Scientists later found that serum antibodies in the blood of survivors of the 1918–19 pandemic neutralized the ability of the swine flu virus to agglutinate red blood cells. (The evidence that the 1918 pandemic was caused by the swine flu virus, while reasonably convincing, was certainly not proof.)

On Valentine's Day, 1976, a day after the identification of the Fort Dix virus as one resembling the agent of swine influenza, a number of concerned scientists had assembled in Atlanta to discuss the swine flu problem. They agreed that no publicity should be given to the Fort Dix outbreak until its significance—whether the harbinger of a pandemic or isolated event—could be assessed. Unfortunately, it soon became clear that uninformed leaks to the press had occurred.

On ABC Evening News on Thursday, February 19, Harry Reasoner made a thirty-second announcement on the existence of a variety of swine flu at Fort Dix that resembled the 1918 variety and noted that a CDC spokesman had said that further investigation was required. The next day, Harold M. Schmeck, Jr., a science writer for the *New York Times*, reported on a press conference called in Atlanta by Dr. David Sencer, director of the CDC. Schmeck wrote that the virus "that caused the greatest world pandemic in modern history . . . may have returned." He also quoted Dr. H. Bruce Dull, assistant director of the CDC, who pointed out that "it is possible the cluster of cases at Fort Dix represents little more than a curiosity." That evening John Chancellor devoted two minutes of NBC Evening News to the swine flu story, with pictures from the 1918 pandemic. The Fort Dix virus was described as new and very dangerous. Dr. Dull's comment that swine flu might be merely an isolated incident was also quoted, along with his statement that although no vaccine against swine flu presently existed, one could be made.

Less than a week after the Atlanta meeting, Dr. Sencer called a press conference to set the record straight as best he could. He succeeded. A flurry of reports came soon after the news conference, then the news media lost interest in the story for something more than a month.

The specter of a 1918 type of influenza pandemic presented both an apocalyptic threat and an unprecedented opportunity. Many influenza experts believed, mistakenly as it turned out, that whenever a major change occurred in the flu virus (a so-called antigenic shift, in which large portions of the viral antigens abruptly change, in contrast to the more frequent but less menacing antigenic drift that occurs when a single amino acid in the antigenic molecules is exchanged for another), the result was inevitably a pandemic. The change would produce a new strain, to which no one could be expected to have any significant immunity. If A/New Jersey/76 had the virulence of the 1918 strain that it so closely resembled antigenically, the resulting "excess deaths"—the number of deaths above those expected from ordinary causes—could run into the hundreds of thousands. In the 1957 Asian flu pandemic there were 70,000 "excess deaths" in the United States, and nearly half that many eleven years later when the Asian flu virus (H_2N_2) went through an antigenic shift to become Hong Kong flu (H_3N_2). Hong Kong flu afflicted more than 50 million Americans, and cost the nation some $4 billion in lost earnings and medical costs.

The cost in lives, dollars, and social disruption of a repeat of the 1918–19 pandemic was incalculable. But was the threat of such a recurrence real? Not everyone thought so. The hinge on which the argument turned was the one-to-one relationship between major changes (antigenic shifts) in the influenza virus and the appearance of pandemics. But the evidence supporting this view was extremely limited.

By 1976, there had been just three influenza pandemics in the twentieth century; in 1918, 1957, and 1968. Thus unimpeachable evidence for the dictum that pandemics follow antigenic shift as night follows day rested on a grand total of two pandemics (1957 and 1968) that had occurred since the isolation of influenza viruses became possible.

A member of the editorial staff of the *New York Times*, whose sharp words would continue to pierce the flesh of those involved in the swine flu program, wrote in a February 23 editorial: "The experts of the Federal Government's Center for Disease Control have raised the possibility—and it is only that—of a worldwide influenza pandemic on the scale of the 1918–19 disaster. . . . It is no light matter to frighten people that such devastation may be repeated, especially when these alarms have been sounded on the basis of tenuous evidence. . . ."

But if the threat were real, the opportunity it provided in the field of public health was even more unusual. Because of the extraordinarily early appearance of swine flu in 1976, public health officials could consider producing a vaccine against it that would be available before the 1976–77 influenza season (roughly November through March). Gearing up for large-scale vaccine production takes four to six months. Under the usual circumstances, when a new influenza variant is identified only a few months at most before the beginning of the epidemic season, the option of large-scale vaccine preparation is not available. In 1976, it was a tempting possibility.

Less than a month after the identification of swine flu at Fort Dix, the CDC's Advisory Committee on Immunization Practices (ACIP) met in Atlanta to consider the magnitude of the threat that swine flu represented, and the measures that might be taken against it. At this point, there had been no further cases of swine flu other than the cluster at Fort Dix. *New York Times* writer Harold Schmeck brilliantly described the ACIP's dilemma when he later wrote, on March 21, "It was as though they had heard a single scream in the night and then silence."

On Wednesday, March 10, 1976, five weeks after David Lewis's death, the ACIP made its recommendation. The committee proposed that a vaccine should be produced against A/New Jersey/76 and plans made to administer it. The ACIP did not, however, recommend mass immunization.

Prior to the 1940s, public health physicians and scientists were at the forefront of society's battle against infectious disease. Since there were few or no effective treatments for such diseases as plague, smallpox, typhoid, and yellow fever, emphasis was rightly placed on preventing epidemics by combinations of vaccination, sanitation, and quarantine. In the 1940s, the rapid development of antimicrobial drugs (which coincided with the development of potent insecticides and rodenticides) changed all that. For the first time it was possible to cure many of the most frightful of the infectious diseases. Death rates from tuberculosis, diphtheria, and typhoid dropped precipitously, and, aside from the decade-long campaign against poliomyelitis beginning in the mid-1950s, the spotlight shifted away from the seemingly pedestrian preventive medicine to the more dramatically effective treatment of hitherto virtually untreatable diseases. By 1976 it had been many years since the public had waited with bated breath for an announcement from an official of the U.S. Public Health Service about the latest disease menace to confront them.

Perhaps Dr. David Judson Sencer, fifty-one, the quiet, hardworking, hard-driving, and dedicated director of the CDC, was caught up by the same excitement that had surrounded the 1950s breakthroughs. Possibly he was overly swayed by the eloquent arguments of one of the more persuasive proponents of mass influenza vaccination. Whatever the reason, Dr. Sencer, three days after receiving the ACIP's report, fired off an "action memo" to President Gerald Ford recommending that every one of America's 213 million people be vaccinated against swine flu.

The memo rocketed upward through the bureaucracy— the assistant secretary for Health, the secretary of Health, Education, and Welfare (HEW), the Office of Management and Budget, and the Domestic Council—before landing on the president's desk. Sencer noted that there was "a strong possibility that this country will experience widespread A/ swine influenza in 1976–77," and pointed out that "the Administration can tolerate unnecessary health expenditures better than unnecessary death and illness."[1] At that point it seemed an either/or proposition—either unnecessary death and illness or unnecessary health expenditures. It was not yet clear that the country could have both unnecessary health expenditures and unnecessary death and illness simultaneously.

The memo went on to suggest that Congress would act if the president didn't; it invoked the memory of the 1918–19 epidemic that killed "more than 400 of every 100,000 Americans"; and it proposed a mass immunization program that would cost the comparatively modest sum of $134 million. After a discussion of the Sencer memo, the secretary of Health, Education, and Welfare, David Mathews, youthful former president of the University of Alabama, sent a note to James T. Lynn, director of the Office of Management and Budget. Mathews stated: "The projections are that this virus will kill one million Americans in 1976."[2] This was a slightly exaggerated extrapolation of the casualty rate in 1918–19 as given in Sencer's memo; but no one had suggested that anything like such a rate would occur in 1976.

Then, eleven days after Sencer had completed his memo, President Ford met in the White House with a team of advisers (assembled on forty-eight-hours notice, and dominated by stout proponents of vaccination), to discuss the Sencer memo. The meeting of Wednesday, March 24, began at 3:30 P.M. in the Cabinet Room overlooking the Rose Garden and the flowering crab apple trees surrounding it.

After hearing individual speakers present their views, the president solicited comments from others around the mahogany table as their aides and associates listened intently from leather armchairs set against the walls. Then he asked for a show of hands as to whether he should take the action recommended in the Sencer memo. Portraits of former presidents looked down impassively as all hands went up. Late in the afternoon the president adjourned the meeting, after telling those assembled that he would wait for a few minutes in the Oval Office at the corner of the West Wing if anyone wanted to express doubts to him privately. How privately such doubts might be expressed when the doubter would have to leave the Cabinet Room under the eyes of his colleagues was open to some conjecture.

When no one came to the Oval Office, the president returned to the Cabinet Room, collected scientific superstars Drs. Jonas Salk and Albert Sabin from among those assembled, and marched to the Press Room over the old swimming pool. There the assembled reporters had been reading a "Fact Sheet" on swine flu handed out even while the meeting in the Cabinet Room was in progress. Now President Ford, flanked by Salk and Sabin, announced his support for a program to immunize "every man, woman, and child in America," and his intention to ask Congress "to appropriate $135 million, prior to their April recess" for vaccine production and administration.[3]

It was a daring proposal. In the 1960s, some 100 million Americans had received oral polio vaccines in an eighteen-month period. Dr. Sencer's aim, espoused by the president, was to vaccinate twice that number in something like ninety days beginning in July.

Many of the participants in the Cabinet Room meeting that preceded Ford's announcement felt, with good reason, that the outcome had already been decided upon before they were summoned; their role was to provide the trappings of democratic process. Some of them said so, and added their voices to those of the critics who had not been invited to assemble in the West Wing of the White House. As Robert Pierpont of CBS News said that evening, "Some experts seriously question whether it is logistically possible to inoculate two hundred million Americans by next fall. But beyond that, some doctors and public health officials have told CBS News that they believe that such a massive program is premature and unwise, that there is not enough proof of the need for it, and it won't prevent more common types of flu. But because President Ford and others are endorsing the program, those who oppose it privately are afraid to say so in public."[4]

True to his word, Ford sent to the Congress, just forty-eight hours after his announcement, his administration's request for a $135 million supplemental appropriation for a national program of immunization against A/New Jersey/76. Congressional reaction was prompt. Paul Rogers's subcommittee on Health and the Environment held hearings on the president's bill on March 31. Dr. Theodore Cooper, assistant secretary for Health, and Dr. Sencer's boss, testified that the Fort Dix virus "has been noted to be similar, quite similar, to the agent that probably caused the 1918–19 epidemic." His prepared statement was equally cautious: "The strain detected among Fort Dix recruits is related to the swine flu virus which has been implicated as the cause of the 1918–19 epidemic."[5]

On April 5, Mr. Rogers brought the bill to the floor of the House. After recognition by the Speaker, he intoned the ancient parliamentary formula, "Mr. Speaker, I yield myself such time as I may consume," then launched into a thorough and careful discussion of the bill. He described the new virus strain as similar to that which caused the 1918–19 pandemic, but went on to say that "The new strain cannot be said to be the same as that which caused the 1918–19 epidemic because the virus which caused that epidemic is no longer available. . . . It should be noted that while this new flu is similar to the Swine flu that caused the 1918–19 pandemic, nobody can say whether or not it would be as virulent as that one since its identification with the earlier one is only partial."[6] The honorable gentleman from Florida had obviously done his homework.

Not everyone had. Ten days after Mr. Rogers's speech to the House, at 1:50 P.M. in the Oval Office, the president signed the bill creating Public Law 94-266, which authorized the program he had requested. Mr. Ford stated, "This virus *was* the cause of a pandemic in 1918 and 1919 that resulted in over half a million deaths in the United States" (italics added). Later he said, "I intend to give this program my direct attention and support because the health of our Nation is at stake."[7]

The legislative history of the bills authorizing the National Influenza Immunization Program (NIIP, or NIP for short) provided an amazing demonstration of the speed with which Congress can act on those rare occasions when it finds it desirable to do so. Defenders of the Congress against the customary charges of sloth and indolence could point with pride to the progress of P.L. 94-266. Or could they?

Fort Dix, New Jersey, is a vast cluster of wooden and one- to three-story rectangular brick buildings set in monotonous rows on flat, treeless ground with virtually no landscaping. The effect is severe, functional, and depressing. Fort Dix is remarkably devoid of charm even by the modest standards of military installations. More important, in April 1976, it was also devoid of swine flu; it had been since a few days after the death of David Lewis. There was influenza, a lot of it, but it was entirely A/Victoria/75.

Swine flu had unquestionably appeared at Fort Dix and been communicated from person to person. The isolation of training companies from one another, especially during the first four weeks, made the epidemiology of swine flu at Fort Dix unusually clearcut and convincing. The swine flu epidemic had overlapped a concurrent epidemic of A/Victoria/75 that put the two flu viruses in competition for victims in the same population. And A/Victoria/75 had won. The ferocious swine flu, putative scourge of the world in 1918–19, had simply disappeared from Fort Dix, and A/Victoria had reigned supreme. Moreover, swine flu was generally a milder disease than that caused by the Victoria virus. David Lewis would probably have lived, the critics said, had he followed instructions and stayed in his barracks. Whether this was true or not, swine flu did not seem to be living up to its reputation in the news media as the great killer flu.

But even a small federal program, once launched, is hard to stop. The swine flu program rolled invincibly onward, even though the disease it was designed to combat had inconsiderately chosen to disappear.

The program was beset with confusion. On April 2, Dr. Sencer introduced the director of the CDC Bureau of State Services, Dr. Donald Millar, as manager of the proposed flu immunization program that was still being debated in the Congress. A week later in Washington, Dr. Cooper of HEW conferred the same title on Dr. W. Delano Meriwether, a hematologist on the Public Health Service staff. Sencer was furious, but could do nothing; the order had come directly from HEW Secretary Mathews to Cooper. "The trouble was,"

Dr. Sencer said later, "that Cooper was looking for work; he had nothing much to do. . . . That Administration had stifled all initiatives. The place was at a dead stop."[8]

Critics of the immunization program had a field day. At a WHO meeting in Geneva, influenza experts from sixteen countries argued that the Fort Dix cluster of swine flu cases could have been an "isolated event," and that there was no evidence of an epidemic. The group recommended that countries prepare vaccine for high-risk groups and wait for further developments. This was duly reported by Walter Cronkite on the day after the president's announcement that he would seek an appropriation for NIP. From Washington, George Herman of CBS interviewed Dr. Sidney Wolfe, director of Ralph Nader's Health Research Group, who deplored the government's scare tactics. The following evening, John Chancellor of NBC raised the question of a political motive for the swine flu vaccination program and NBC reporter Lee McCarthy in Atlanta made the practical point that the cost of eggs was certain to rise because of the requirement for some 100 million eggs for vaccine production.

On April 6, the *New York Times* published another scathing editorial. It began: "President Ford may—or may not—have considered, at least for a fleeting moment, the political dividends of being seen as the savior of the American people's health when he decided to call for a $135 million rush program to vaccinate every person in this country." The editorial went on to express doubts about the basic assumptions underlying the program, namely: the danger of swine flu in 1976–77; whether vaccine production and administration could be accomplished in time; the effectiveness of the vaccine; and whether the benefits exceeded the costs, "in terms of human distress as well as money." The writer then wrapped himself in a prophet's cloak and made the accurate prediction: "It is conceivable that if there is no flu epidemic . . . a not inconsiderable number of people might suffer harmful effects with little or no gain." The column ended with a searing sentence: "The President's medical advisors seem to have panicked and to have talked him into a decision based on the worst assumptions about the still poorly known virus and the best assumptions about the vaccines."

On April 22, an article appeared in the *New York Times* by Dr. John S. Marr, head of New York's Bureau of Preventable Diseases, and Gwyneth Cravens, a contributing editor of *Harper's*, in which they discussed the financial and temporal restraints on the swine flu immunization program as it affected New York City. They pointed out that the federal government was appropriating about 10 cents per immunization, while the cost would be at least five times that. None of the states had that kind of money in their public health budgets, in the authors' view, and neither did New York City. Moreover, considering the number of immunization centers in the five boroughs of the city and their hours of operation, it would require one year, not ninety days, to immunize New York's 8 million people (to say nothing of the 1.5 million illegal aliens and 6 million commuters who made up the city's total daytime population). The same point about the cost of vaccine administration had been made in congressional testimony by the president of the Association of State and Territorial Health Officers, Dr. Eugene Fowinkle, who estimated the cost of administering the shots at 50 to 70 cents each. At the same hearing, Constance Hollerman, R.N., speaking for the American Nurses Association, pointed out that to meet the president's goal, 1 million persons would have to be vaccinated every day, seven days a week, for six months.

On the day before Marr and Cravens's piece appeared, a little drama, described by one critic as pure Monty Python,[9] was played out in the crowded eleventh-floor lobby of the National Institutes of Health (NIH) Clinical Center (a 500-bed hospital) in Bethesda, Maryland. Diminutive Theodore Cooper, M.D., of HEW administered a swine flu shot in the left arm of Harry M. Meyer, Jr., M.D., director of the Bureau of Biologics of the Federal Drug Administration (FDA), who towered over him. A few minutes later, amid jollities for the audience and the television cameras, Dr. Meyer gave the needle to Dr. Cooper (like Goliath hurling a stone back at David), while in an adjoining room the same injection was being given to 200 volunteers from NIH and FDA. The following week similar trials would begin in Rochester, New York, and Houston, Texas.

Both Dr. Cooper and Dr. Meyer emphasized at the Clinical Center ceremony that "At present no one can guess the probability that the swine flu virus will emerge next winter as the main cause of flu in the U.S."

Dr. Cooper, trained as a cardiac surgeon, was an early ally of David Sencer. He respected Dr. Sencer's expertise in the matter of communicable diseases, and Cooper's father, also a physician, had told him ghastly tales about 1918–19. Theodore Cooper became Sencer's most effective medical supporter in Washington, since he was highly regarded by influential members of Congress as well as by key people in the administration.

Harry Reasoner brought videotapes of the NIH ceremony to NBC viewers that evening, while Jim McManus of CBS also interviewed an FDA commissioner, Dr. Alex Schmidt, who pointed out that "no one will get swine flu from eating pork chops unless they also kiss pigs."

In late May, the *New Yorker* ran a short piece entitled "Swine Flu Over the Cuckoo's Nest" that chronicled an interview with a fictional Rhinehart Glanzerman, described as a pathogen press agent and influenza impresario. According to the writer of the piece, Richard Liebmann–Smith, the swine flu virus had received nearly every major prize given by the American Academy of Medicine, carrying off "coveted 'Jonases' for Best Disease, Best Symptoms, Best Virus, Best Potential Epidemic. . . ." "It's beautiful," Glanzerman said. "With two hundred million vaccinations booked for next season, we're out-inoculating Polio, Measles, and Smallpox combined." In the course of the interview, Glanzerman held up a newspaper that announced the medical profession's support for massive flu vaccination in terms modeled on *Variety's* inimitable headlines: "QUAX BACK MAX VAX!"

"How did Swine Flu make it big?" asked the interviewer. "I played the nostalgia angle," Glanzerman replied. "These last few seasons have all been revivals anyway, and I figured the Swine was a natural. . . ." Whether the author of the *New Yorker* story had Dr. Sencer in mind as a model for his epidemic entrepreneur is unknown, but comparisons, however odious, were widely drawn between the energetic R. Glanzerman and the controversial director of the CDC.

There were more serious criticisms as well. The *New York Times* loosed another editorial arrow on June 8: "President Ford may not know it; but with each passing day the . . . swine flu immunization program appears less necessary and more unwise." The writer pointed out that there was no swine flu anywhere in the world and that no other nation was emulating the U.S. campaign, "while a significant number of advanced industrial countries are just shrugging the whole thing off as one of those incomprehensible American abberations and over-reactions that appear occasionally in election years." The next day, the *Times* carried a report from Geneva by Walter Sullivan, who wrote that the European health specialists were questioning the American program because of the risk of serious side effects. In these experts' view, he wrote, "The program can only be justified if the risk of a serious outbreak is substantial."

There were other problems. What of the possibility that A/New Jersey/76 would undergo another antigenic shift before the 1976–77 flu season, rendering the 200 million doses of vaccine useless? What if the expected epidemic never appeared at all? After all, the swine flu virus, in its A/New Jersey/76 form, had not shown itself to be either particularly lethal or robust. And what about side effects? Was it really safe to vaccinate pregnant women and young children, or older children for that matter? No vaccination, even with physiological saline, is ever totally without side effects if enough people are given it. And if 213 million persons were to be vaccinated, some of them would certainly suffer serious, possibly permanent, injury. As CBS Evening News quoted Dr. Martin Goldfield of the New Jersey Health Department on April 2, "There are as many dangers to going ahead with immunizing the population as there are in withholding. We can soberly estimate that approximately fifteen percent of the entire population will suffer disability reactions." This "sober estimate" was, in fact, grossly inflated, but the problem was nonetheless real.

Who was liable for such disability? Was it the vaccine manufacturers, the distributers, the physicians, nurses, or technicians giving the injections, the federal government, or all of the above?

The point of vaccine efficacy was also a bone of contention. Dr. J. Anthony Morris, then director of the slow, latent, and temperate virus section of the Bureau of Biologics, stated: "If it were up to me, I wouldn't even start making the vaccine. There is no clear-cut evidence that inactivated [killed] influenza vaccines offer appreciable protection to the recipients."[10] Dr. Morris, who was ultimately fired from his job with the FDA, claimed that his dismissal was because of his opposition to the swine flu program, although the FDA's action against him had begun years before.

Another group of critics of the NIP suggested stockpiling the vaccine in case a swine flu epidemic began, as the other industrial nations had done. This procedure would weigh the certainty of side effects from a mass immunization program against the likelihood of a swine flu epidemic: if no epidemic occurred, mass immunization would be unnecessary.

Three government agencies involved in the mass immunization program were responsible for answering these questions of risk and benefit. The CDC, because of its statutory role in disease control, was at the spearpoint of the campaign. Responsibility for passing on all licensed vaccines rested with a little known agency, the Bureau of Biologics, formerly part of the NIH but now part of the FDA. The program of administering the vaccine to volunteers and tabulating the results fell to another branch of NIH, known as the National Institute for Allergy and Infectious Diseases (NIAID). The Bureau of Biologics and NIAID were nearly neighbors in the northern Washington, D.C., suburbs, while the CDC was 600 miles south in Atlanta. This arrangement carried the seeds of a public relations disaster; seeds that would soon sprout into hideous flowers.

Public relations catastrophes were not new to vaccine programs, as the transfer of the Bureau of Biologics from NIH to FDA probably indicated. That apparently political move happened in 1955, after a newly developed vaccine against poliomyelitis was rushed onto the market and led to 10 deaths and 192 cases of paralytic polio among recipients of the vaccine and their families because the virus was not effectively inactivated (killed) by the manufacturer (Cutter Laboratories of San Francisco). The Cutter vaccine incident caused the resignation of a secretary of HEW, a surgeon general, and a director of the NIH. It was a bit of history that kept popping into the minds of those in charge of the swine flu immunization program.

Meanwhile, the scientists and administrators continued with the intent of beginning vaccination in July. The influenza experts were well aware that, in 1918, the full-blown pandemic had begun in August. On May 7, the CDC Advisory Committee on Immunization Practices met again in Atlanta, and, according to Harold Schmeck in the *New York Times*, "The experts seemed unanimously agreed that the project should proceed," although Dr. E. Russell Alexander, a highly regarded influenza expert from the University of Washington, Seattle, suggested that a final decision on vaccination should depend on whether there was further evidence that the Fort Dix virus was affecting people elsewhere. He had written to Dr. Sencer earlier "to say once more that I strongly recommend some hesitation before beginning vaccine administration. . . . I do not agree that it [vaccine administration] need necessarily be carried out, unless there is another swine outbreak."[11] Later,

Alexander expressed his philosophy more fully in an interview: "My personal view is that you should be very conservative about putting foreign material into the human body. . . . If you don't need to give it, don't."[12]

In a Manhattan laboratory, work on developing a vaccine strain of the swine flu virus had begun in February as soon as the organism had been recognized. Edwin M. Kilbourne, M.D., is head of the Department of Microbiology at the Mount Sinai School of Medicine, a recognized expert on influenza, and editor of a widely used textbook on the subject. A trim, handsome, blue-eyed, and bearded man who looked much younger than his fifty-six years, Kilbourne was one of the NIP's staunchest supporters. He had attended the White House meeting on March 24 that preceded President Ford's announcement of his support for the NIP.

The laboratory work was carried out by Barbara Pokorny, a small, vivacious, dark-haired woman who had been Dr. Kilbourne's assistant for twenty-one years. She first candled fifty-four fertilized eggs by holding them against a strong light, which allowed the chick embryos and associated blood vessels to be clearly seen. Barbara Pokorny put a pencil mark on each egg where injection could be made without hitting a blood vessel. Using an electric drill equipped with a dental burr, she then made holes in the small end of each egg, so that the internal pressure caused by later injection would not burst the shell. Then, with a diamond-pointed stylus designed for marking on glass, she quickly chipped away the shell under the pencil mark and injected samples of the swine flu virus. The eggs were incubated in a warm room just down the hall from Pokorny's laboratory, in the Annenberg Building sixteen stories above Central Park.

It was only sensible to assume that there was considerable risk of infection with the new agent, and Barbara Pokorny was told not to tell anyone what she was doing. As she said later, "I wouldn't let anyone in the lab. They really thought I had flipped out."

After the initial batch of eggs had been incubated long enough to yield substantial quantities of virus, the small ends of the eggs were cut off with a special tool (a circular, spring-driven blade) and the virus-containing amniotic fluid removed and tested. Later, Pokorny inoculated other eggs with both the swine flu virus and a laboratory strain of influenza virus (known as PR 8) that does not grow in man but grows rapidly in eggs.

The purpose was to create a new virus from the mixture of PR 8 and the swine flu virus. Viruses are basically genetic material (DNA or RNA, which encode an organism's individual traits), surrounded by a protein sheath. Different viruses, when mixed together, are capable of exchanging pieces of their genetic material (genes) to produce new strains that bear a mixture of the traits of the "parent" viruses. The resultant offspring viruses are known as recombinants. In Pokorny's experiment, the genes of the two viruses would recombine in the egg. If only two properties were considered—possession of the H_{1sw} antigen from the swine flu virus, and the capacity for rapid growth of the laboratory strain—the recombinants would fall into four groups. Two of the four would be identical to the parental viruses: the slow-growing swine flu virus and the fast-growing PR 8. The other two would be new: a fast-growing swine flu virus and a slow-growing PR 8.

The next step was to separate the PR 8 virus from the swine flu strains. If hemagglutination antibody to PR 8 were added to the mixture of viruses, PR 8 would be neutralized as the antigen-antibody complex, leaving behind only the different swine flu viruses. Repeated inoculation into eggs and collection of this pair of viruses rapidly enriched the egg fluids in the fast-growing recombinant strain of the swine flu virus. The latter, because of its superior growth rate, rapidly became the dominant population. Thus eventually all the PR 8 strains were eliminated, leaving only the swine flu viruses.

The desired recombinant strain, which could be grown quickly to produce the necessary vaccines, was labeled X-53. On the weekend of February 27, it was sent to Dr. Francis

Ennis of NIAID and to the CDC. The executives of one drug company were so anxious to start vaccine production that they sent a messenger to Dr. Ennis's home in Bethesda that weekend to pick up a sample of the seed virus. (A sample of seed virus given to the manufacturers a week earlier had grown poorly in eggs; Kilbourne's recombinant solved that problem.)[13] Analysis of X-53 showed that six of its eight genes came from PR 8, and two genes, for the hemagglutination and neuraminidase antigens, were contributed by the swine flu virus.

The role of a vaccine is to trick the body into thinking it has been infected by the disease in question so it will manufacture antibodies against the foreign organism that will enable the body's defensive system to recognize and destroy it. With influenza, the production of disease is a two-step process. In the first step, the invading virus (the term "virus" is from the Latin word for poison) attaches to cells in the upper respiratory tract of its victim. This attachment constitutes infection with the virus, which does not necessarily lead to disease. Viral attachment to cells in the nose, mouth, and throat of its host depends upon the hemagglutination antigen on the surface of the flu virus, and is prevented by antibodies to the viral H protein. The second step after infection is the development of disease as the virus spreads from cell to cell, destroying them and releasing substances from the damaged and dying cells that result in the headache, fever, and weakness associated with influenza. The spread of the virus from cell to cell depends on the neuraminidase antigen of the viral coat. In fact, neuraminidase may play a major role in determining viral virulence. Thus the body's second line of defense against influenza is the production of antibodies against the viral N antigen. Kilbourne's recombinant, with its H and N antigens from PR 8, was ready for vaccine production.

In the fall of 1918, swine influenza had first appeared as a new disease in pigs in the Midwestern United States. Over the next few months millions of animals were sick and tens of thousands died. Veterinarian Dr. J. S. Koen of Fort Dodge, Iowa, an inspector for the U.S. Department of Agriculture, noticed the coincidental new illness in humans and swine; it was he who christened the disease in pigs "swine influenza." To this day a milder form of swine flu appears in pigs in every state, but particularly in the Midwest, each fall and winter. Further investigation led scientists in the influenza field to conclude that the swine virus that first appeared in humans in 1918 continued to circulate in man for another eight or ten years. And there was evidence that flu viruses could pass from humans to pigs.

Although swine flu virus was isolated from five human cases in Czechoslovakia in 1960, it was 1974 before the virus was found in a human being in the United States. The victim was a fourteen-year-old boy, who died at the Mayo clinic in Rochester, Minnesota, from Hodgkins' disease. He had been in contact with pigs just a few days before his death. But once the disease had disappeared from Fort Dix, there were no other cases to be found anywhere.

Dr. Kilbourne was quoted as saying in late March, "Our thought is that probably the virus is seeded in foci around the country, and when winter comes we will see it again."[14] The fact that swine flu had apparently disappeared didn't particularly disturb the experts. The Asian flu epidemic of 1957 had begun as an isolated outbreak in Iowa, then died out. After a second flurry of cases in Pennsylvania, the virus disappeared as suddenly as it had come. It was two months before the full-blown Asian flu pandemic began to appear.

Canadian health authorities carefully considered the situation, then arranged for production of enough vaccine (from laboratories as far away as Australia) to protect half the Canadian population, particularly those at high risk and those carrying out essential services (doctors, nurses, and firemen, for example). At the federal level, the Canadian government considered and rejected the stockpiling option, although three of the ten provinces (Quebec, Manitoba, and British Columbia) elected to postpone administering the vaccine until the need for it was demonstrated. In England, the Advisory Group on Influenza saw no need for mass immunization and chose instead to have a United Kingdom firm make 1 million doses of the vaccine (for a population of about 56 million) to immunize high-risk groups. Soviet authorities let it be known that they would prepare the vaccine but would stockpile it against the possibility of a pandemic.

But U.S. experts were preparing for mass immunization to combat the expected eruption of swine flu. It would take some days to publicize the need for vaccination and set up the facilities (even assuming that all the machinery was in place and waiting). Ten days to two weeks would be necessary before those immunized would have significant levels of protective antibody against A/New Jersey/76. By then, it might be too late. In 1918–19, after all, previously healthy adults had sickened and died in twenty-four hours. The position of most of the American public health establishment remained what it had always been—full speed ahead for the National Influenza Immunization Program (NIP).

Meanwhile, 6 or 7 million pigs were being trundled off to market each month. The pigs were no strangers to swine flu; many of them had had it and, like humans, they coughed, ran fevers, breathed with difficulty, and even fell prostrate, seemingly on the very brink of death. There was a certain amount of ham in these pitiful piggy performances. Fewer than one in a hundred pigs ever died of swine flu, although those that died were usually the younger animals, and a few pregnant sows aborted when they contracted the disease. The biggest problem was a temporary loss of weight. That was really the pig farmer's problem, since it meant that the swine would have to be fed longer before being sent to market.

Seven million pigs is a lot of pigs. If 7 million pigs marched single file into a Chicago stockyard, they would form a line of swine reaching at least from Chicago to Moscow via London. And, sure enough, someone noticed all those pigs.

If, indeed, American pigs were the repository of the virus that caused the 1918–19 pandemic, some experts asked, then why not vaccinate them and wipe out the disease at its source? The question was first raised at a Bureau of Biologics influenza workshop the day after President Ford's announcement of his support for the NIP, then at a WHO meeting in Geneva two weeks later. It came up again at a Department of Agriculture meeting in Hyattsville, Maryland, in early May.

For the pig producers represented by the National Livestock and Meat Board, this suggestion was absolutely the last straw. They were already upset over the name "swine flu"; they had recurring nightmares about the sale of pork plummeting as people got the idea that they could get influenza from eating pork chops or bacon. The Board argued, quite reasonably, that the name of the virus strain should reflect, by hallowed tradition, the place where it was discovered. It should, they said, be called "New Jersey flu," instead of swine flu. The state of New Jersey, through Governor Brendan Byrne, respectfully declined the honor.

The Livestock Board viewed swine flu as a disease that people gave to pigs, rather than the other way around, and the idea of porcine vaccination was anathema to them. And the prospect for successful vaccination of the pigs was not encouraging. Hog cholera, a far more serious disease than swine influenza, could have been eradicated completely, yet not even half the pigs had been vaccinated because the pig producers would not cooperate. What chance, then, had vaccination for the relatively innocuous swine influenza?*

Meanwhile, on June 4, 1976, the CDC issued a preliminary statement on influenza vaccine outlining the reasons for proceeding with NIP and discussing the further vaccine trials for efficacy and safety that were to begin shortly. Then,

---

* Hog cholera was virtually eradicated late in 1976 by the simple expedient of testing herds and then slaughtering every animal in a herd in which an infected pig was found.

The Perilous Voyage of the Good Ship NIP: Triumph and Tragedy

The underwriters who handled liability coverage for the four drug firms making swine flu vaccine had been nervously communing with their computers ever since Public Law 94-266, which launched the National Influenza Immunization Program, had been signed in mid-April 1976. By early June the massed transistors—the modern equivalent of the Delphic oracle—had spoken. The actuaries had asked: Can we cover the vaccine companies against claims resulting from the NIP? The computers replied: No way! Or better, that the risks involved could not be computed and therefore could not be insured against.

The jaws of four drug company presidents dropped in unison when that word came from their friendly local insurance agents. The insurance company actuaries predicted claims in the billions of dollars resulting from the statistically inevitable incidence of side effects, mostly trivial, but some very serious. As Leslie Cheek of the American Insurance Association said later, "The courts have turned the tort system into a compensation system. If someone dies after receiving a

shot the attitude is, 'He's dead. Let's give him some money.' "[1]
Giving money to a corpse may have seemed a bit odd, but
Cheek's point was clear enough to vaccine makers: no drug
company could absorb costs of that magnitude and survive.
The four drug company presidents, in the finest tradition of
American free enterprise, promptly turned to Washington for
help. It was a simple syllogism. The government wanted the
vaccines. The companies couldn't afford to make the vaccines
without insurance against lawsuits resulting from their administration. Ergo, the government should provide the insurance.

A telegram sent on June 15 from the chairman of the
board of one drug company, Warner-Lambert, to the president, members of Congress, and various federal officials gives
the flavor of the argument: "I must call your attention to the
impossible situation that has been created by the sudden withdrawal yesterday by our insurance carrier of our liability insurance for your swine flu program. Our company is more
than willing to produce the vaccine for the Government
program. However, we are placed in an untenable position . . .
without any insurance coverage or other liability protection."[2]

All the vaccine manufacturers were in the same boat; their
insurance would be withdrawn on July 1, and all urged passage
of legislation permitting the government to assume liability.
The government's initial reply was the same as that of the
actuaries' computers: No way! After sober reflection, the
relevant committees of Congress also chorused—No way! The
good ship NIP was dead in the water and leaking badly, and
it soon became clear that no one was going to be immunized in
July or even August.

In retrospect, the most surprising thing about the liability
issue is that anyone was surprised. Maurice Hilleman, the
head of virology for the drug company Merck, Sharpe, &
Dohme, and a member of the panel that had convened at the
White House on March 24, had raised the liability issue years
before. And in January 1976, as the flu virus was just beginning
to raise its swinish head at Fort Dix—before it was identified

as a potential problem—Dr. H. Bruce Dull of the Center for Disease Control (CDC) had prepared a staff paper on the subject of liability that was routed from Sencer to Cooper to Mathews, head of HEW. The covering memo pointed out that "Manufacturer liability for vaccine-associated disability . . . threatens a predictable vaccine supply. . . ."[3]

On April 13, two months before the telegram from Warner-Lambert, the *New York Times* noted that "the drug industry has expressed concern over the question of liability," and went on to quote a statement by a Merck spokesman and by Joseph Stetler, president of the Pharmaceutical Manufacturers Association. The Senate Appropriations Committee, after passing the supplemental appropriations bill establishing funds for the NIP, noted: "The Committee explicitly directs that the various governmental units shall be free from liability . . . for the vaccine, its quality, and any adverse reactions directly attributable to the vaccine. . . ."[4] Also on April 13, John J. Horan, president of Merck, had written Mathews, eleven congressmen, and five government officials that Merck had been warned by its insurer that coverage for the swine flu vaccine was "not feasible at virtually any price."[5] Now everyone acted as if the issue of liability had never occurred to him.

Part of the problem may have been that Dr. Theodore Cooper wanted to avoid issues where physicians were subordinate to, and hence at the mercy of, lawyers. (Or, as one of Cooper's close associates put it, "Doctors think lawyers are a pain in the ass. Cooper's mind set was to keep lawyers out if you don't want it screwed up.")[6] But lawyers could hardly be blamed for the disaster of the liability issue.

The third week in June 1976 was a bad week for the immunization program. Parke-Davis & Company had contracted to produce nearly half the total amount of vaccine required for the program. They had geared up quickly for production runs ten times the normal size, and, with commendable industry, had already produced some 6 million doses by the middle of June. But one third of them were of a vaccine against the wrong virus. Parke-Davis had on hand some 2 million doses of vaccine against the organism isolated from pigs by Richard Shope—in 1930! They might have been wonderfully effective in 1918, but this was 1976 and the virus of interest was A/New Jersey/76. How had the mix-up occurred? No one was saying much. Spokesmen for HEW said that Parke-Davis had obviously used the wrong virus strain in part of its production. Parke-Davis denied this, and hinted that A/New Jersey/76 had changed its characteristics as type A influenza viruses are wont to do. Dr. Harry M. Meyer, Jr., of the FDA said only that production control techniques were being tightened to ensure against a repetition of the calamity. The clear implication was that they were something less than tight before.

It's important to note that the same batch of seed vaccine virus went from Dr. Kilbourne's New York laboratory through HEW to all four vaccine manufacturers, but only Parke-Davis made the wrong vaccine.

On July 2, Dr. Dull of CDC was quoted by the *New York Times* as saying at a meeting in New York's Americana Hotel that there was no reason to believe the new swine flu virus would be any more deadly than the other flu strains of recent years. He went on to describe the swine flu virus as a human flu virus with the H antigen of the swine virus attached to it, and pointed out that testing had shown that the H antigen was not responsible for the severity of the 1918–19 pandemic. Then Dr. Sidney Wolfe of Nader's Health Research Group made this prophetic remark: "The major disease in the U.S. this year related to Fort Dix will not be swine flu but, rather, swine flu vaccine disease."

An editorial in the *New York Times* the next day reviewed the problems of vaccination with the swine flu vaccine, then commented: "Behind these developments is growing skepticism at every level about the scare propaganda used originally to jam the relevant legislation . . . through Congress last spring." The editorial concluded: "President Ford should take the lead in modifying the swine flu program to a more modest and reasonable level, and in abandoning the frenzied emergency program that scaremongers foisted on the nation."

Then, the Monday after Independence Day in the glorious Bicentennial Year of 1976, the embattled NIP came under fire from what it might have thought were friendly batteries. Albert Sabin, M.D., developer of the attennuated (live) polio virus that had largely supplanted Salk's inactivated vaccine in the United States, and who had stood at President Ford's elbow as Ford announced his proposal for the NIP, told the House Subcommittee on Health and the Environment what he had told a professional meeting in Bethesda two weeks before: "It is evident that the original plan for mass vaccination of every man, woman, and child in the U.S.A. as a means of preventing a potential epidemic of swine influenza virus disease is no longer possible."[7]

Although the first clinical trials of the vaccine (on over 5,000 volunteers) had shown that the vaccine from all four manufacturers—Merck, Sharpe, & Dohme; Merrill-National Laboratories (a subsidiary of Warner-Lambert); Parke-Davis; and Wyeth Laboratories—gave good antibody response in people over twenty-four with mild side effects in two out of every hundred vaccinees, only the Merck vaccine gave adequate antibody response in a large proportion (73 percent) in those between seventeen and twenty-three, and in children six to ten in whom it also produced a substantial incidence of accompanying fever. Only half the children three to six years of age had an adequate antibody response to either the Merck or Merrill vaccine; the vaccines from the other two manufacturers were almost totally ineffective.[8]

The subcommittee sat in stunned silence as Dr. Sabin pointed out that if only the adult population were inoculated, the virus would spread broadly enough in children so that an epidemic could be expected in 1977. By then, immunity would be lost. He called for consideration of the plan to stockpile vaccine and administer it only if further cases occurred. Actually, Albert Sabin had had some doubts about influenza vaccines all along. He had written Dr. Sencer on the eve of the March 24 White House meeting to say: "I am impressed by the number of reports of studies on young adults in the army, insurance company employees, etc. in which the use of potent influenza vaccines had failed to make a significant impact on the total incidence of acute respiratory disease. . . ."[9]

Dr. Kilbourne of Mount Sinai School of Medicine then admitted to the subcommittee that the Fort Dix outbreak could have been a "freak occurrence." He could hardly have said otherwise, since he had described the NIP in print as "A $135 Million Gamble."[10] And that's what it clearly was, except that far more than $135 million was actually at stake. Dr. Kilbourne and most of his colleagues thought that the risk was only that the $135 million might be wasted if an epidemic of swine flu never occurred. The possibility of substantial deaths—or disability—as a consequence of the NIP was not then appreciated.

Drs. Salk and Cooper strongly defended the NIP before the congressmen and they carried the day. Jonas Salk spoke as he had earlier at the Bethesda meeting of storing doses of vaccine in people rather than in warehouses. Subcommittee chairman Representative Paul G. Rogers (D-Fla.) continued his vigorous support of the mass immunization program.

Television networks suddenly took an interest in the stockpiling issue and featured that odd couple Dr. Albert Sabin—still as lively in his early seventies as when he left his native Russia as a boy in 1920—and mild-mannered Dr. E. Russell Alexander. Sabin, who describes his former status as that of "white-haired boy"—the walls of his corner office on the second floor of the Basic Science Building, Medical University of South Carolina (Charleston), were covered with pictures of him with Presidents Johnson, Nixon, and Ford, beside the records of many other honors—now found himself at cool remove from his former colleagues, and especially from David Sencer. Dr. Alexander was similarly treated.

A week after the subcommittee hearings, the CDC's Advisory Committee on Immunization Practices (ACIP) issued detailed recommendations on matching the various groups of people involved with an almost bewildering array of vaccines. The NIP would provide a vaccine only against A/New Jersey/76. Since it contained only one variety of antigen, it was called monovalent. Two of the four manufacturers were making whole monovalent virus vaccine against A/New Jersey/76; two others were splitting the virus into its antigenic protein coat and the viral genetic material (in this case RNA, or ribonucleic acid). Only the antigenic protein went into the vaccine. There were also whole and split versions of a monovalent vaccine against B/Hong Kong/72, and of a bivalent vaccine against A/New Jersey/76 and A/Victoria/75. Obviously, the list did not include all possible combinations, but it was complex enough.

The whole virus preparations gave a better antibody response but produced somewhat more side reactions. For the high-risk group, the ACIP recommended administration of the bivalent swine flu and A/Victoria vaccine, to be followed some days later by the monovalent B/Hong Kong vaccine. Pregnancy was not considered a bar to immunization, although the question of what to do about people under eighteen was put off until the results of further tests were available.

The ACIP mentioned reports of rare neurological disorders and even deaths associated with vaccination against influenza. From the millions of influenza vaccinations administered in nearly a quarter of a century had come only a dozen reports of consequent neurological disease, and only three reports of fatal illness—all in people at substantial risk of death even in the absence of influenza vaccination. Since the vaccine was grown in fertilized hens' eggs, it would contain traces of egg protein. Therefore people allergic to eggs could not receive the vaccine, but this only involved 1 person in 100,000, and even they could be desensitized if they chose to be.

In mid-July, the Washington *Star* reported that the Armed Forces Epidemiology Board refused to endorse the vaccines made by Wyeth and by Parke-Davis for administration to military personnel for the reasons that Sabin had out-lined for the Rogers subcommittee. And on July 20, the *New York Times* launched another editorial attack on the NIP: "With the passage of time, there has been increasing incongruity between the panic measures advocated by President Ford . . . and the reality. . . ." The writer quoted a British medical school professor, Sir Charles Stuart-Harris, physician and author of a respected textbook on influenza: "It is indeed highly questionable whether the amount of vaccine required . . . should be prepared at the present time for any country, including even the United States, until the shape of things to come can be seen more clearly." The *Times* editor went on to charge that "the relative paucity of similarly plain-speaking expert voices in this country" was due to the politically charged atmosphere of an election year and the dependence of medical researchers on federal money. This unfortunate statement cast aspersions on the integrity of all biomedical scientists in the United States while ignoring the fact that their counterparts in England and elsewhere were at least equally dependent on government support for their research activities.

As July gave way to August, some 120 million doses of influenza vaccine had been produced but remained un-processed for distribution because of the liability problem. Merrill-National Laboratories, which had produced nearly half of the total by this time, had stopped production entirely. Congress refused to act on a bill allowing the government to assume liability for damages arising from the NIP, and there had been no other cases of swine flu anywhere in the world, although rumors abounded. Then eighteen persons died of a mysterious ailment while attending an American Legion convention in Philadelphia in July (see chapter 7), and the press speculated that the cause might be swine flu. There were false reports of hundreds of deaths from swine flu in Australia, along with cases in the Philippines and Taiwan that received wide newspaper and television coverage.

Meanwhile, the British were saying pish, tush, and pooh

to swine flu. Six volunteers were deliberately exposed to the disease and, as reported in the British medical weekly *The Lancet* on July 3, they suffered only mild illnesses and the induced influenza did not spread to others. Charges and countercharges continued to fly. Dr. Cooper stated that government experts were agreed that "in recent years flu vaccines have been up to 90 percent effective when the infecting virus matches the virus used in the vaccine."[11] But Dr. Sidney Wolfe, head of Ralph Nader's Health Research Group, considered influenza vaccines "clearly less effective than other vaccines with efficacies running from twenty to seventy percent."[12] Despite Cooper's assessment, some government experts sided with Wolfe, while others admitted privately that the effectiveness of any given flu vaccine could be anything from zero to 100 percent depending on how and by whom the tests were made.

By mid-August, the question of immunizing children was not yet settled. School-age children from five to fourteen are usually considered to be the prime spreaders of influenza. If they could not be vaccinated, as Dr. Sabin had pointed out to Representative Rogers's subcommittee, there was nothing to prevent an epidemic from breaking out.

Of course, it is no surprise that in an election year there would be charges that President Ford had declared war on swine flu as a means of demonstrating his concern for the public's health. Critics pointed out that, until the outbreak at Fort Dix, President Ford's interest in public health had been principally manifested in his repeated vetoes of appropriation bills for the Department of Health, Education and Welfare (the parent agency of the National Institutes of Health, the Public Health Service, and the Center for Disease Control). There was not a jot of evidence, however, that Ford's support for the NIP, no matter how hastily marshaled, had been primarily politically motivated.

Politically, the swine flu vaccination program was a no-win situation. If a swine flu pandemic arrived, then nothing that the Ford administration had done would be enough. If it did not arrive, then those who had been vaccinated in vain would be painfully reminded of it as they raised their sore arms to the voting booth levers. John Cochran of NBC News had smelled a political rat somewhere in the hold of the good ship NIP even before it was launched, and he thoroughly canvased Ford's political advisers for confirmation of his suspicions. He was unable to find anyone who was enthusiastic about the program. Cochran therefore concluded that Ford's motivation for sponsoring the immunization program could not be political.[13]

There were only two clear-cut groups of winners in the NIP sweepstakes. As NBC reporter Lee McCarthy pointed out, one group was America's chicken farmers, who found that the demand for fertilized eggs used in vaccine testing had soared after several years of declining egg consumption brought about by fear of dietary cholesterol. And America's roosters, faced with an unprecedented challenge, had risen to it with the fervor of true patriots. As Earl Butz, secretary of Agriculture, had put it in late March: "The roosters of America are ready to do their duty. . . ."

It was becoming increasingly clear that there would be two malignant results from administering the swine flu vaccine. First, there would be the inevitable serious reactions leading to permanent injury or death. The percentage would surely be small, but even a minuscule percentage, when multiplied by 100 million people, or however many might actually receive the vaccine, would lead to an impressive number of serious side effects. It was also clear that the vaccine program would lead to a transient rise in such things as the lead poisoning and rat bites that occur mostly in slum children, and in venereal disease, since the funds and the personnel whose job it was to deal with these problems would be temporarily siphoned off to help with the swine flu immunization.

Meanwhile, in Philadelphia 26 persons had died by early August and 175 more were hospitalized with the mysterious disease that was thought, briefly, to be swine flu. The highly publicized threat coincided with the decision of Congress in mid-August to pass the bill making the federal government liable for any illness resulting from the swine flu vaccine under the Federal Tort Claims Act, which sets legal fees at a much lower than average rate, eliminates jury trials and punitive damages, and encourages out-of-court settlements.

This sudden resolution was aided by the fact that Congress was scheduled for one of its frequent adjournments in mid-August, this time for the Republican National Convention. As Representative Tim Carter, M.D., of Kentucky put it: "This is no time to banter about legalism, but it is time to act on behalf of the public health of the United States." This view was by no means unanimous. Representative Henry Waxman said: "I feel more and more uncomfortable the Federal Government is going to be stuck for the whole tab."[14] And later, Representative Waxman accused the drug companies of attempting to blackmail the federal government, while in the Senate, Edward Kennedy charged that the insurance companies were "failing to assume a responsible posture."[15]

The bill that finally passed permitted the federal government to sue drug companies, or the groups administering the vaccine, if they were considered to have been negligent. The manufacturers promptly negotiated a pool with more than forty insurance companies to underwrite a $220 million package to protect them against governmental suits for negligence. With the impasse over liability broken, vaccine production could resume and the vast quantities of vaccine already made and stored in bulk could be bottled in usable form.

There was a great sense of elation among many of the scientists and administrators of the immunization program when the indemnification bill was signed by the president on August 12. Now the good ship NIP could get under way again, and all hands rushed to raise the sails. Their enthusiasm was premature. Under congressional budget procedure, the legislation would not become effective until October 1, the beginning of the new fiscal year, and the vaccine suppliers were certainly not going to permit anyone to be immunized before then.

By the time the roadblock of indemnity had been cleared away, it was widely recognized in the scientific community that the influenza vaccines failed to produce antibody to neuraminidase. Thus the body's primary defense against influenza infection (antibodies against the H antigen) would be stimulated by the vaccine; but those virus particles that escaped these antibodies and attached to the cells in the upper respiratory tract could readily spread from cell to cell and produce disease without inhibition by antibodies against the N antigen.

This deficiency of the vaccines had actually been noted in a report given by Dr. Alan P. Kendal of the CDC at a meeting at NIH on June 21, but the word had spread only slowly. Dr. Kendal's tests of the seed strains used by the manufacturers showed that they contained ample neuraminidase activity, suggesting that the N antigen had somehow been lost during production!

But what difference did it make? As Dr. Kilbourne, who produced the vaccine strains, put it: "It would obviously be desirable to have a vaccine that raised the antibody to both neuraminadase and hemagglutinin."[16] No one knew for certain what the effect would be on vaccine potency, but informed guesses suggested a loss of activity of some 10 to 20 percent. Those deeply involved in the NIP showed only mild concern, but as a scientist for one of the manufacturers explained it, "What else could they say? We've got 150 million doses of vaccine without neuraminadase. That has to be their stand."[17]

Another irony, in a program festooned with ironies, was that the "wrong" vaccine made by Parke-Davis before the error was corrected had neuraminidase, and its hemagglutinin, while not a perfect match for A/New Jersey/76, did stimulate antibody production that would have some effect on the swine flu virus. So it was possible that the "wrong" vaccine, with two active antigens, might be more effective than the "right" vaccine with only one. If anyone in the scientific community still believed that the experts had a detailed understanding of influenza and influenza vaccine production, they might equally well have believed in "creation science" and Laetrile.

Dr. W. Delano Meriwether, the thirty-three-year-old hematologist and Olympic-class sprinter who was managing the NIP, spoke to the Washington Press Club on August 11 and said that the target date for beginning immunization was late September (the fact that the program couldn't start until the beginning of the new fiscal year was still not widely appreciated). This was already two months behind schedule. Dr. Meriwether pointed out that to vaccinate even half of the population by the end of December would require a million immunizations each day.

By October 1, only about a quarter of the vaccine originally expected was on hand, thanks to the delay engendered by the liability controversy. There could never be enough vaccine to immunize more than 70 percent of the adult population. If shots for those under eighteen were ever recommended, the vaccine deficiency would be even greater.

There was yet another foul-up. The original deadline for accepting vaccine deliveries by the government was December 3. In the third week in September, government officials advised the vaccine manufacturers that they would accept deliveries for another six weeks beyond the original deadline. But one of the manufacturers had already stopped production to avoid having vaccine coming out of the plant after the December 3 deadline! Since it would take ninety days to produce the first additional batches of vaccine from the shutdown facilities, it was obviously pointless to restart them. Meanwhile, a Gallup poll taken at the end of August showed that only 53 percent of Americans intended to be vaccinated against swine flu; 17 percent did not intend to be vaccinated; and the remaining 30 percent were uncertain.

Dr. Cooper of HEW was certain that vaccination would begin in early October and that well over 100 million vaccine doses would be distributed between then and Christmas. In an interview late in September, he denied rumors that the vaccine could produce influenza in a recipient. This could have happened with an attenuated (living) viral vaccine, or with an inactivated viral vaccine in which the inactivation step was only partially successful (as in the 1955 Cutter incident); but both the manufacturers and the Bureau of Biologics were very careful to ensure that it would not happen. As Dr. Cooper described the vaccine, "This is as high a quality product as could be made available to the public."[18] That somewhat Delphic pronouncement was intended to assure the American people that the vaccine was the safest ever made, which it probably was, but the statement was open to a variety of interpretations.

Cooper also responded vigorously to the liability question: "The insurers did not say that the vaccine wasn't medically safe. What they were saying is that because this was a highly visible, publicly supported program, there could be baseless lawsuits that could potentially cost billions of dollars.

"That's an incredible, irresponsible prediction. There is absolutely no reason to think of a number of suits of that dimension."[19] There was nothing Delphic about that statement. But events were to prove that the actuaries were right and Dr. Cooper was wrong, even though his view was supported by thirty years of influenza vaccine history.

In 1976, for the first time, the CDC had the money to set up an elaborate and sensitive surveillance system, directed by Dr. Michael Hattwick and manned around the clock seven days a week to detect and record side effects from the swine flu vaccine. Such effects had undoubtedly occurred in previous vaccination campaigns but had gone unnoticed in the absence of a sophisticated system to uncover them.

Still, the cost of the Hong Kong influenza epidemic in 1968–69 that had led to 50 million cases of the disease in the

United States, and to some 33,000 "excess" deaths, was estimated at nearly $4 billion in medical expenses, lost working
days, insurance paid to survivors of the deceased, and so on.
If the NIP prevented even a fraction of such a loss it was, at
a mere $135 million, an excellent investment. One group of
scientists estimated the economic benefit of the NIP using a
computer analysis of educated guesses appropriately called the
Delphi technique. They concluded that the vaccination of
those over twenty-five was economically justified only if 59
percent of the people in that group accepted immunization,
if the cost of producing and administering the vaccine was 50
cents, and if the probability of an epidemic was 10 percent.
Expert estimates of the probability of an epidemic ranged
from 2 to 25 percent, so a 10 percent chance was a reasonable
average.[20]

In early October, the National Influenza Immunization
Program finally got under way. The complexities of the immunization plan were evident in the New York City program.

Pascal James Imperato, M.D., known to his friends as
Pat, was appointed chairman of the New York Swine Influenza
Task Force early in April. It was a big job and there wasn't
much time. Originally, the intention was to begin immunizing
high-risk groups in July (with the bivalent vaccine against both
A/New Jersey/76 and A/Victoria/75), then in September
begin giving the monovalent vaccine against swine flu to the
rest of the population over eighteen.

In New York City, ninety new employees, all college
graduates, were hired and trained to use the automatic jet
injectors capable of administering 1,000 shots an hour with
which much of the vaccine would be given, and also to give
cardiopulmonary resuscitation if necessary. Seventy-five sanitary inspectors and 150 public health nursing assistants were
similarly trained. Five or six hundred volunteers were recruited
through the Red Cross for each day the immunization program was to last, and forty-five immunization clinics were
established throughout the city, supplemented by fifteen

mobile teams to inoculate people in nursing homes and senior citizen centers. Sixty teams of six persons each were set up. Each team included a supervisor, two vaccinators, and three clerical and support personnel.

Each vaccine recipient was to receive an information sheet (available in English, Chinese, Japanese, Italian, Yiddish, French, Spanish, and Greek) explaining the advantages of immunization, the risks involved (as they were understood at that time), and giving telephone numbers in each of the five boroughs that could be called in the event of a severe reaction. Each vaccinee also had to sign a consent form stating that he or she agreed to the immunization after reading of its benefits and risks. Along with all this, a public education program was conducted using radio, TV, and local newspapers.

New York City had some 6 million people above the age of eighteen. The city was promised 10 million doses of vaccine; it received 4 million. The federal grant money to New York City for its portion of the NIP was approximately $3.5 million. This covered the cost of the vaccine (about $2.1 million), nearly $1 million in personnel costs, the purchase of eighty jet injectors (at about $1,000 each), and other supplies and travel expenses. In addition, the New York City Department of Health spent more than $1 million from its own budget in support of the swine flu immunization program, and this meant curtailing or suspending other Department public health activities.[21]

The impressive capacity of the jet injector for rapid immunization was largely wasted. It was like using a Ferrari to deliver milk. The rate-limiting step in the program was the speed with which the vaccinees could read the information sheets and informed consent forms. In spite of all difficulties and months of delay, however, the New York City portion of the NIP got under way with the ceremonial opening of one of the sixty immunization stations at 9:00 A.M. on Tuesday, October 12, 1976. Pat Imperato got his shot from a volunteer at the Lower Manhattan Health Center at 303 Ninth Avenue.

Attendance at the clinics was excellent. That first morning in New York City some 15,000 people were successfully vaccinated and Dr. Imperato could take justifiable pride in the outcome.

Then the NIP suffered another frightful blow. During the opening ceremonies of the immunization stations in New York City, both Associated Press (AP) and United Press International (UPI) reported that three persons had died in Pittsburgh, Pennsylvania, following swine flu vaccination the previous day. Before the day was out, Alaska, Illinois, Louisiana, Minnesota, Maine, New Hampshire, New Mexico, Texas, and Wisconsin had suspended the immunization program and the telephone switchboards at the CDC, Atlanta, were threatening to melt under the heat of incoming calls from frantic public health officials from one end of the country to the other asking what had happened in Pittsburgh.

What had happened in Pittsburgh happened at the Pittsburgh health department's South Side clinic, a one-story brick building at 1016 East Carson Street that served many of the workers in the nearby steel mills and their families.[22] On the fateful day, clinic personnel were immunizing high-risk people with batch number 913339A bivalent vaccine from Parke-Davis & Company; 1,242 high-risk persons were immunized at the South Side clinic that day. Of that number, there were five serious reactions.

The first was a sixty-four-year-old woman who became pale, weak, and dizzy after immunization. Although the clinic's nurses called an ambulance for her, the woman refused to go to the hospital. Instead she was escorted home, and when contacted the next day, was back to normal.

The second serious reaction occurred in a seventy-five-year-old woman, Mrs. Julia Bucci, who had a history of heart and lung problems, hypertension, obesity, and diabetes. She was only able to reach the clinic with the support of her husband and daughter and a tripod cane. Within minutes after receiving the injection (a disposable syringe and needle were used instead of the jet injector because, although slower, they cause less pain and tissue damage), Mrs. Bucci said she felt weak. She became pale, her lips turned blue, and she had difficulty breathing. Nurses gave her oxygen and called an ambulance. By the time it arrived, she felt better and was talking to people as she was being put into the ambulance. She died an hour after arriving at the hospital from arteriosclerotic heart disease and acute pulmonary edema.

The next reaction took place in an eighty-one-year-old woman who had angina pains earlier that morning and had taken two nitroglycerin tablets before going to the clinic. This woman became faint while Mrs. Bucci was being put in the ambulance. She was revived with ammonia inhalant and also taken to the hospital. She was examined in the emergency room, found normal, and sent home.

The second and third victims of fatal reactions were a seventy-one-year-old man, Charles Gabig, and seventy-four-year-old Ella Michael, both of whom left the clinic without any signs of ill effects from the immunization after the compulsory fifteen-minute waiting period. Mr. Gabig went shopping with his wife after leaving the clinic, but complained of pains in both arms while they were in the grocery store. He immediately went home and lay down. He was found dead shortly afterward of a heart attack, a blood clot, and other cardiovascular problems.

Ella Michael had a history of cardiovascular disease and emphysema. She, too, died at her home that afternoon, some six hours after the immunization. Autopsies on all three of these elderly persons revealed nothing unexpected in the light of their known ailments. A telephone survey of more than 10 percent of those vaccinated at the South Side clinic that day failed to turn up additional serious reactions, nor did the area's hospitals report admission of other heart attack victims who had recently been vaccinated.

The Pittsburgh coroner, Cyril H. Wecht, had degrees in both medicine and law and a reputation for flamboyance as a result of his persistent and highly publicized attacks on the Warren Commission's investigation of the assassination of President John F. Kennedy. Wecht came prancing before reporters and TV cameras to claim that federal and state health officials, presumably including the CDC team that arrived in Pittsburgh from Atlanta at 3:20 A.M. the morning after the deaths, had dismissed the possibility "that something went wrong." Dr. Wecht, after looking at a television film clip of immunizations given at another clinic and at a different time, claimed that the nurses giving the injections weren't pulling back on the plunger before depressing it to ensure that they were not giving the vaccine directly into the bloodstream. Experts quickly dismissed this allegation as absurd.[23] (Competent nurses pull the plunger of a hypodermic syringe back as a matter of course, with a movement too subtle to be seen readily on a TV film clip.) In any case, Dr. Wecht might profitably have spent a few minutes with his copy of *Gray's Anatomy*. There are no significant blood vessels in the deltoid muscle of the upper arm where the injections were given. Had there been any, the needle was too short to reach them; and even if a blood vessel had been penetrated, there was no reason why death should ensue since the vaccine had been given intravenously to animals without effect.

Later, Dr. Wecht wrote that the NIP had been suspended nationwide because of the Pittsburgh deaths, which was not true, and that the investigation of those deaths by CDC personnel "was nothing short of a whitewash."[24] Dr. Wecht left it as an exercise for the reader to determine what such a whitewash might accomplish in view of the merciless publicity that surrounded the NIP.

Careful investigation of the vaccine itself, and of the circumstances under which it was administered, failed to demonstrate a causal relationship between the deaths and the swine flu vaccine. In New York City, after a midday emergency meeting of the city's Department of Health, the staff recommended continuing with the immunization program although the bivalent vaccine being used for high-risk patients was the same batch as that used in Pittsburgh's South Side clinic.

From a public relations standpoint, however, the fat was in the fire. Headlines in the New York City newspapers the following day screamed: "The Scene at the Death Clinic," and "Death Toll Mounting." The *New York Post* described Mrs. Bucci's death as follows: She "had winced at the sting of the hypodermic . . . taken a few feeble steps, then dropped dead." That was not what happened, but it didn't seem to matter. The *New York Times* page 1 headline stated simply: "Swine Flu Program is Halted in 9 States as 3 Die After Shots." The subheading explained that no evidence was found to show that the deaths were the result of the vaccination. But the damage was done. Attendance at immunization clinics plummeted. Although 15,000 people had been inoculated in New York City on the first morning, the rate subsequently fell to an average of 5,000 a day.

At the CDC that terrible Tuesday, while radio and television were spreading rumors about the Pittsburgh incident, tempers were growing short. Dolores Frederick, science and medical writer for the *Pittsburgh Press*, described the atmosphere: "The public information person [at the CDC] kept saying I would have to use the wire services because the information was given to them. After considerable verbal pressure the public information person was cajoled into putting me in touch with some higher-up public information officials. But even then they cut me off quickly so that the questions I had weren't really answered." One anonymous reporter who got through to Dr. Donald Millar at the CDC described him as "abrasive, pompous, and antagonistic." It's possible that Dr. Millar felt the same way about the reporter. And Thomas O'Toole, science writer for the Washington *Post*, labeled the CDC as the most "offensive" of all the government agencies he had dealt with.[25]

Dr. Imperato's staff in New York City was unable to reach anyone at the Center for Disease Control; his public health colleagues around the country had the same problem. As Dr. Imperato later wrote: "Had the Center acted promptly and decisively, they might have forged a unified position across the country."[26] As it was, nine states suspended vaccination, others stopped using the vaccine batch in question, and some, like New York City, went ahead as planned on the assumption that for three elderly ill persons to die within six hours of one another after sharing a common traumatic experience (vaccination at the South Side clinic) was almost certainly not of any statistical significance. Unfortunately, by the time the CDC finally came out with a statement, it was too late to avoid a public relations crisis.

On Thursday, October 14, Gerald and Betty Ford, son Jack, and daughter Susan assembled with the White House physician and a battery of television cameras in the basement of the mansion to receive their swine flu shots, and business at the immunization centers picked up somewhat, although Jimmy Carter, Ford's rival for the presidency, refused the immunization. Walter Cronkite came close to apologizing on his radio show for the conduct of the various news media. He said: "The qualifiers [in a catastrophe story like this one] never quite seem to repair the damage done by the initial statement. . . . The repetition of stories which appeared to link death and vaccination have spread the damage like wildfire."[27]

At that point, fourteen people had died within forty-eight hours of receiving flu vaccine and a *New York Times* editorial on October 14 opined that "President Ford will be well advised to order a halt in the vaccination program." The editorial failed to mention that the average age of the fourteen victims was slightly over seventy-two years, and that all but one of them had a history of heart disease.

The next day, Dr. Millar of the CDC pointed out that, since the launching of the NIP on October 1, 1 million persons over sixty-five had received swine flu shots; out of that 1 million, thirty-five people had died within forty-eight hours of vaccination. But, as Dr. Millar noted, out of 1 million persons over sixty-five, 160 could be expected, on average, to die each day, nearly half of them from heart disease.[28] Dr. Millar's data were reassuring, though disputable. In retrospect, however, it would have been far better to have made these facts clear to the medical profession, to the Congress, and to the people before the NIP was launched. Failure to do so had led to the second catastrophe (after the liability flap) in the NIP's short and troubled life.

An illuminating survey of the media coverage given the swine flu program during the catastrophic week that began with the deaths in Pittsburgh was later published in the *Annals of Internal Medicine*.[29] The authors, Dr. David Rubin and Val Hendy of the Department of Journalism of New York University, found newspaper coverage generally to be voluminous, reasonably accurate, and exceedingly superficial because of most reporters' lack of scientific background. In total coverage the newspaper of record, the *New York Times*, led the pack of the nineteen daily newspapers surveyed by Rubin and Hendy, with an imposing 320 column inches (fifteen articles) devoted to swine flu. The Miami *Herald* was close behind. At the other end of the spectrum was the Denver *Post*, serving a county of half a million population (in 1970), and offering only 61 column inches on swine flu, with almost a third of the total in a single story. Even the Casper *Star-Tribune* (of Wyoming; county population, about 40,000 in 1970) did better than the Denver *Post*, which is generally considered to be the major newspaper of the Rocky Mountain West. But the Denver *Post* itself looked good compared with television, whose coverage was superficial even by poor newspaper standards. The one third of Americans who rely exclusively on television for their news were (and probably always are) very poorly informed indeed.

Eleven days after the deaths in Pittsburgh, the U.S. Public Health Service finally recommended vaccination of three- to seventeen-year-olds, with two inoculations four weeks apart.

Split virus monovalent vaccine was to be used in healthy people from three to seventeen, and either split or whole virus monovalent vaccine for healthy people over seventeen. Split virus bivalent vaccine was recommended for high-risk individuals between three and seventeen years, with a booster a month later. High-risk children six months to three years old were to get the same vaccine and booster at half the dose, while whole virus bivalent vaccine was to be used for high-risk individuals aged twenty-five to sixty-five, and in all those over sixty-five. If a harassed public health officer found that battery of proposals confusing, he was not alone. The recommendation of four different vaccines to different age groups, two of which required a booster after four weeks, had the ring of nightmare. It was virtually impossible to administer such a complex program to tens of millions of people in two months time.

Meanwhile, much of the press seemed primarily concerned with body counts, since they were unprepared to discuss the scientific and medical aspects of the program. One UPI reporter was forced to explain to his superiors why, at one point, AP had a higher body count than UPI. Nervous UPI clients demanded an explanation.[30]

The NIP, severely wounded by its public relations disaster, poor planning, simple bad luck, and unrealistic recommendations, staggered along through the remainder of October and most of November without much additional excitement. Then, on November 23, 1976, Larry Hardison, father of two, a thirty-two-year-old lineman for the Continental Telephone Co. in Concordia, Missouri, awoke and, in Lord Byron's phrase, found himself famous.

Deserving though the town may have been, the world had not often turned its gaze toward Concordia, Missouri (population 1,850). But in mid-October, Larry Hardison contracted a fever, sore throat, and cough. His physician, Dr. Jerry Meyer, took a blood sample and sent Hardison home to bed for a few days. Nearly a month later, Dr. Meyer took another blood sample and sent it off to the state health department laboratory. The results in the state laboratory were confirmed by the CDC. Larry Hardison had developed swine flu antibodies in the month between blood samples. When Larry Hardison went to work on Monday, November 23, the television cameras were waiting and pictures of the rather baffled young man in a hard hat and sideburns down to his chin wafted out over the airwaves.

From the standpoint of NIP proponents, Larry Hardison and his apparent case of swine flu had come along at just the right time. Even though the evidence was not wholly convincing since the virus had not been isolated from him, he was the closest thing to a swine flu victim that had appeared in 1976 since the death of Private Lewis. The NIP plan was to immunize some 150 million adults by the end of the year. New Year's Eve was five weeks away and only 25 million people had received the swine flu vaccination. In fact, on the day the news about Larry Hardison went out, Dr. Meriwether announced a campaign of posters, newspaper messages, and radio and television commercials to publicize the NIP, sponsored by the Advertising Council and managed by the firm of Altman, Stoller, & Weiss at no cost to the federal government.

The campaign theme was: "Get a Shot of Protection. A Swine Flu Shot." One sixty-second TV spot described how a handsome mustached young man named Joe brought swine flu home from the office and gave it to his wife, Betty, one of his kids, and to Betty's mother who was visiting from California. The next day Betty's mother flew home and transmitted the disease to her best friend, Dotty, who had a heart condition and died from complications of swine influenza.

For a brief time, however, Larry Hardison was worth more to the NIP than a dozen TV spots. In New York City, after the report from Concordia, the Health Department switchboard was jammed by inquiries for vaccine information —30,000 calls came in, of which only 5,000 could be answered. It was the same in Missouri and elsewhere. As a gently ironic touch, Larry Hardison had to break off his interviews with reporters to install two extra telephone lines in the Health Department office in Concordia's City Hall.

Meanwhile, back in New York City, the number of daily immunizations rose from 5,000 to 12,000 under the impact of the news about Larry Hardison; but it soon fell again. By mid-November, fewer than 5 percent of New York City's target population had been immunized. The city's Health Department then conducted a survey among middle-class commuters and the inner-city poor. Over 60 percent of the commuters thought the immunization was unnecessary; less than 20 percent were afraid to be immunized. Less than half the inner-city poor thought the vaccination was unnecessary, but nearly 40 percent were afraid of the shots.

About the same time a CDC spokesman charged that the large city programs were failing to reach black and other minority populations. This certainly did not apply to New York City, where most of the flu clinics were housed in public health buildings built in the 1930s and 1940s in what, by 1976, had become inner-city poverty areas. The statement also assumed that the urban poor wanted to be immunized, a questionable assumption in light of the New York City survey.

In late November and early December, two cases of swine flu were confirmed by isolation of the virus from the victims, both in Wisconsin, and both in people who had had close contact with pigs. But the public was becoming blasé about swine flu and reports of these cases did not stimulate the market for immunization.

On December 10 what many public health officials had feared all along was confirmed. Dr. Lyle Conrad, assistant director of the immunization division of the CDC, was quoted in an AP dispatch as noting that there had been 36,375 cases of measles in the United States by November 22, compared with 22,754 cases at the same time a year earlier—an increase of 60 percent. Dr. Conrad added that the expected increase would be even greater the following year, in part because of the diversion of public health resources to the swine flu program. "It has diverted attention and time and personnel and money from immunization for other diseases, including measles," he said.[31]

Meanwhile, back in Washington, Theodore Cooper enjoyed a splendid office on the seventh floor of the spanking new HEW building on Independence Avenue. But the magnificent office had, more often than not, resembled a sort of medieval torture chamber, and not only because the roof leaked when it rained. The long hard battle to bring the NIP to a successful conclusion had taken its toll. Now, with Christmas Eve just ten days away, the final blow fell that would put the National Influenza Program forever out of its misery.

On Tuesday, December 14, CDC officials announced that they were investigating reports that at least thirty persons in ten states had developed paralysis after receiving the swine flu vaccine. The ascending paralysis, most often called Guillain-Barré syndrome from the names of the French doctors who first described it in 1916, had also occurred in twenty-one persons who had not received the vaccine. Since Guillain-Barré syndrome (or GBS) was not a reportable disease, the CDC had little information on the normal incidence of the malady, which was also called French polio.

Two days later the NIP was suspended, supposedly temporarily, until the matter of GBS could be cleared up. By that point there were ninety-four cases of GBS reported from fourteen states. Fifty-one cases, and all of the fatalities, had occurred in people who had received swine flu vaccine.

On the television evening news programs the next day, the cancellation of the NIP was a big story; NBC, for example, devoted almost six minutes to it. Walter Cronkite reported the 107 cases of temporary paralysis on CBS. Edwin Kilbourne was interviewed in New York and offered his reason for thinking that GBS and the swine flu vaccinations were unrelated, namely, that GBS had been around for years and that there was no proven relationship between the disease and vaccination. David Brinkley and his colleagues interviewed Theodore

Cooper, who said that the GBS problem would take several weeks to pin down. Michael Hattwick, M.D., the man in charge of the CDC's surveillance network, was surprised that there were so few reactions being reported to the vaccination. The TV news programs aired a shot of a woman at a CDC switchboard telling a caller that 90 percent of GBS victims recovered. Inevitably, Dr. J. Anthony Morris, who had earlier questioned the efficacy of the vaccines, pointed out that it had been known since 1966 that influenza vaccination was a factor in eliciting GBS and that he had been fired from the FDA because of his opposition to the swine flu program. Neither statement was quite true.

In that 1966 paper, the author, Felix Leneman, M.D., of San Francisco, reviewed 1,100 cases of GBS reported in the French, English, and American medical literature between 1950 and 1965. Of these 1,100 cases, only 1 was found to be related to immunization with influenza vaccine, while 8 were due to laboratory-diagnosed influenza A or B infection, and 83 apparently resulted from nonspecific fevers and influenzal syndromes. Thus the risk of contracting GBS subsequent to an influenza infection was much higher than the apparent risk of contracting the disease from flu vaccination.[32]

As for Dr. Morris's oft-repeated claim that he was fired from the FDA because of his role as a "whistle-blower" on the swine flu vaccination program, the charges that terminated in his dismissal in July 1976 were instituted on July 11, 1975. This was after a panel of eight nationally known virologists had agreed, following three days of public meetings in April 1975, that Dr. Morris's performance was unsatisfactory.[33]

By January 31, 1977, 1,098 cases of GBS had been reported to the CDC surveillance center; 532 of the victims had received the swine flu shot before they developed the disease. In both vaccinated and unvaccinated cases, the disease was almost identical; nearly 22 percent (approximately one in four) of the victims in both groups needed mechanical assistance to breathe during the course of the disease, and about 6 percent of those over seventeen died in each group. There were, however, two striking differences between those who contracted GBS after vaccination and those who did not. One difference was in the age distribution; the largest age group in the unvaccinated victims of GBS was 15–19 years, while the vaccinated victims were most heavily represented in the 35–39 age group. So few people age 18 or under received the vaccine that this apparent difference in the age distribution is of questionable significance. The other important difference was in the time distribution of the onset of the paralytic disease. Unvaccinated victims become ill in a random fashion throughout the year, while 71 percent of the vaccinated victims became ill within four weeks of vaccination. The relative risk of acquiring GBS was more than seven times higher in those who had received a swine flu shot than in those who had not. The probability of acquiring GBS after a swine flu shot, however, was only about 1 in 100,000,[34] and is zero in current influenza vaccines (*JAMA*, Aug. 13, 1982).

As the Bicentennial Year of 1976 drew to a close, the great swine flu immunization program, which had stemmed from the death of Private David Lewis on February 4, was finished. With it, perhaps, went the hope of ever again mounting a national immunization program against any infectious disease in the absence of a clearly perceived threat. In all, about 157 million doses of vaccine had been made. More than 46 million civilians had received vaccines through the NIP; military and Veterans Administration programs added 2.5 million more—a total of about 49 million, or twice as many as had ever before been vaccinated in a national campaign.

The *New York Times* editorial writer who had thundered against the NIP from the moment of its inception stepped out from behind the anonymity of the editorial page and revealed himself, in an Op Ed column published on December 21, as Harry Schwartz, a *Times* editorial writer on foreign affairs for nearly three decades. Now he wrote: "Last February and March, on the flimsiest of evidence, President Ford and the Congress were panicked into believing that the country stood at the threshold of a killer flu epidemic."

Among the elements Schwartz cited as contributing to the disaster was empire building by the CDC in order to become "the Government center for health education and disease prevention. Funds used for that purpose inevitably take money away from those whose job it is actually to treat sick people." This view was patently absurd. The Center for Disease Control obviously has as its reason for existence "health education and disease prevention," and, in the last sentence, Schwartz seemed to be saying that it is preferable to treat people after they're sick rather than attempting to prevent their illness in the first place. By what mechanism federal revenues appropriated to the CDC took money away from private physicians was also left unclear.

The day after Christmas 1976, Lawrence K. Altman, M.D., a science writer for the *New York Times*, wrote: "The swine flu immunization program has tarnished, rather than brightened, the reputation of public health in the minds of many people." He added: "Officials now concede that in starting the nation-wide program hastily, they failed to explain the risk possibilities to the public."

Early in February 1977, the new secretary of HEW, Joseph Califano, asked David Sencer to step down as director of the CDC. That action was greeted with cold fury in Atlanta and with a deep sense of unease elsewhere. Dr. Donald A. Henderson, dean of the Johns Hopkins University School of Hygiene and Public Health, and former head of the successful program to eliminate smallpox from the world, reported that news of Sencer's demotion "had resulted in a flood of letters, cables, and other communications . . . from health officials . . . asking what was happening and expressing concern for the Center." In defense of his action, Secretary Califano said that "we got repeated comments [from doctors and public health leaders country-wide] that CDC was not what it once had been and not where it ought to be today."[35]

Early in 1977, the Justice Department reported that it expected to be in litigation over the swine flu program for the next five years. One of the largest claims filed by early February was for $1 million by a man who claimed to have been made impotent by the immunization. At the other end of the spectrum was a woman who claimed that her blouse had been ruined by acetone spilled on it while a clinic worker was cleaning her arm prior to injection.

Under the Tort Claims Act that covered the government's liability, those who considered themselves injured by the swine flu vaccination had to file a claim and allow the government six months to negotiate a settlement before filing suit. The number of claims against the NIP rose steadily. In December 1976, Scott Heath, a twenty-six-year-old Harvard graduate just starting a career as a commercial artist in Denver, filed a claim for $2 million. He received the swine flu shot on November 10, 1976. Two weeks later, he required brain surgery that left him unable to walk, work, or carry on a normal conversation.

In late February, Gary Sabonijan, a twenty-three-year-old electronic technician in New Jersey, filed a $1.5 million claim. In March, Alden S. Adams of Kaysville, Utah, filed a suit for half a million dollars because of partial paralysis following a swine flu immunization. By mid-November 1977, the value of claims against the NIP totaled $2.64 billion. Dr. Cooper had called the actuaries' forecast of lawsuits totaling billions of dollars "an incredible and irresponsible prediction." But the actuaries were right. By then, 2,775 claims had been filed. These included 223 death claims, in addition to personal injury and Guillain-Barré cases. Although the average claim for GBS was $937,203, claims in the other two categories averaged well over $1 million each. The government had paid an average of only $46,000 in the eighteen suits and claims settled by early January 1977.

By late summer 1977, the Justice Department finally settled its first death claim resulting from the NIP. It agreed to pay Kathleen Herbst of Grand Rapids, Michigan, $285,000 for the death of her forty-six-year-old husband seventeen days after receiving the injection. By then, the number of claims settled out of court had risen to seventy-one, but the average settlement had dropped to under $30,000.

The *New York Times* ran an editorial on January 15, 1978, pointing out that there were now 3,700 claimants with claims totaling more than $3.3 billion against the swine flu program and proposing a future no-fault system in which claims would be paid quickly. The writer continued: "Without such compensation, as one critic has observed, the Government is in effect drafting citizens into a war against disease and then telling the injured, 'Thank you for your contribution to the war effort and best of luck in coping with your disability.' "

That's exactly what the government was doing. Five days earlier, the *Times* had reported on the case of Mark Waldvogel, who had been a healthy, athletic high-school senior in Kailua, Hawaii, in 1976. Two weeks after the swine flu shot he became paralyzed from the chest down, apparently from Guillain-Barré syndrome. Now, at twenty, he was paraplegic, confined to a wheelchair for life. As he put it: "It seems only fair that the Government should provide some compensation . . . I can't understand why it's taken so long." At that point only 4 out of 321 GBS suits had been settled and 14 out of 732 claims. By January 1982, the government had paid over $9 million in claims of the more than $3 billion originally demanded.

So the drama of the ill-fated NIP passed from the laboratories and immunization clinics to the courts. Looking back, it is hard to avoid the feeling that the swine flu immunization program was pursued with an almost missionary zeal that led its proponents to ignore obvious problems such as liability, temporally related deaths, and the certainty of some serious side effects, not to mention the complete absence of the disease the NIP was designed to protect against. It was this unswerving determination to carry the program to its planned conclusion, regardless of obstacles and heedless of factors that should have led to reconsideration of its objective, that resulted in the swine flu disaster.

It was not a total disaster, however. Public opinion polls have shown that, although people were highly critical of the swine flu immunization program, they would consider the next call for mass immunization no less favorably than before. Certainly, public awareness of influenza immunization has been greatly enhanced and scientists have learned a great deal about influenza vaccines—dosage, assay, administration, and response—that they could not have learned in a less imposing program. There is also a much more sophisticated view of some of the complications of mass immunization than there was before the NIP. The issues of liability, stockpiling, and possible alternatives to influenza immunization (prophylactic treatment with antiviral agents, for example) have received an intense public scrutiny that can only be beneficial.

Swine flu, or a similar life-threatening illness whose impact can be softened by vaccination, will appear on the American scene some time in the future. Then the lessons of the NIP, if they are not forgotten or ignored, may provide valuable guidance as to what course to take.

4

Toxic Shock

In Rock Hill, South Carolina, on a morning in early October 1980, twenty-year-old Sheila Thompson awoke with a high fever, chills, and a very sore throat. Carolyn Thompson made an appointment for her daughter to see Dr. Robert Lindemann. His diagnosis was that Sheila had a strep throat and he began appropriate treatment, but Sheila's condition grew steadily worse. She became confused and disoriented; her pulse rate rose to twice normal. Twenty-four hours after being seen by the young doctor, she was brought to the hospital emergency room. Two hours later, she was dead. Dr. James Maynard, the pathologist who did the autopsy on Sheila, found a tampon in place. It, and the vagina itself, contained pus and a foul-smelling discharge. Sheila Thompson's life had been taken by Toxic Shock Syndrome, or TSS, now recognized as a fulminating vaginal infection by the bacterium *Staphylococcus aureus*.

CBS Evening News on Monday, October 6, reported Sheila's death and interviewed Dr. Kathryn Shands, a tall, slender woman with brown eyes and shoulder-length brown hair, who was head of the Toxic Shock Syndrome Task Force of physicians and scientists at the federal Centers for Disease Control (CDC) in Atlanta. Dr. Shands cautioned, in connection with Sheila Thompson's death, that it was easy to misdiagnose the disease. Later followed a commercial that Procter and Gamble was exhibiting on 600 commercial television stations at the time. It showed a woman seated at a desk with a package of Rely, Procter and Gamble's brand of tampon, conspicuously displayed beside her. Two weeks before, Procter and Gamble had withdrawn Rely from the market. Now the actress in the TV commercial told women to stop using Rely tampons and to return any unused portion for a refund.[1] Advertisements with a similar message were placed on 350 radio stations and in 1,200 newspapers following the signing by the manufacturer of a consent agreement with the Federal Drug Administration, which has had responsibility for tampons as a "medical device" since 1966. The advertising program would ultimately cost Procter and Gamble some $10 million.

Rely's slogan was "It even absorbs the worry." But, by October 1980, there was far more than the usual worry about tampons in general and Rely in particular. On Friday, September 19, the *Morbidity and Mortality Weekly Report* from the CDC carried a follow-up study on TSS (the *Report* had carried two previous warnings about the disease earlier in the year). The September 19 issue noted that, according to the calculations of CDC experts, women using either Regular or Super Rely had a nearly eight-fold higher risk of contracting TSS than did women using other brands of tampons.

That same day, Procter and Gamble shut down the production lines making Rely in Albany, Georgia, and Cape Girardeau, Missouri. The following Monday, the company recalled Rely from the market, even though its spokesman called the CDC report "too limited and fragmentary for any conclusions to be drawn."[2]

At that point, Procter and Gamble accountants could afford to be philosophical; Rely sales amounted to less than 1 percent of the giant company's annual revenues. The legal branch, however, was not so sanguine. In late August, Linda Imboden, a twenty-seven-year-old mother of three children in Redding, California, had filed a $5 million suit against Procter and Gamble as a result of contracting TSS in May. Most of her waist-length hair had fallen out, clawing of her hands had cost her her dexterity—and her job—and, worst of all, gangrene had destroyed any sensation in her fingertips and two toes. Ultimately, she would lose the tips of some fingers and one toe. Linda Imboden's suit claimed that Procter and Gamble had known of the problems with Rely six months to a year earlier but had given the consumer no warning. Robert Norrish, the public relations director for the company, replied from company headquarters in Cincinnatti that they had only learned of the problem in June.[3]

Also in August, in the San Francisco Bay Area, two teenagers, fifteen-year-old Diana Silva of Livermore and seventeen-year-old Lesa Toby of Vallejo, died of TSS. In late September, a class action suit was filed in San Francisco seeking all the profits Procter and Gamble had made from Rely; a suit in Tucson sought $2.5 million; shortly after Sheila Thompson's death in South Carolina, a $1.25 million suit was brought against Procter and Gamble on behalf of Teresa Commesse, fifteen, of Seldon, Long Island, and Leanne Patierno, twenty-one, of Brooklyn; and a Bronx woman filed a $6 million class action suit against the company. Some 400 suits against Procter and Gamble in connection with Toxic Shock Syndrome were just beginning to come to trial in the spring of 1982. By late April the husband of a twenty-five-year-old mother of two children was awarded $300,000 for her death on September 6, 1980.[4]

These developments received a torrent of attention from the news media. By early October there had been 400 cases of TSS reported to the CDC; Sheila Thompson was the fortieth fatality. There are some 55 million women of menstruating age in America; nearly seven out of every ten used tampons.

Anything that vitally affects the lives of more than 35 million women is naturally a media event.

It's hard to decide when the story of Toxic Shock Syndrome began. That staphylococcal infections may produce toxins leading to life-threatening shock had been known for many years. Cases resembling contemporary TSS were reported as staphylococcal scarlet fever as long ago as 1927, and, in 1978, a Denver pediatrician, Dr. James Todd, and his colleagues reported that they had observed a peculiar disorder in seven children from eight to seventeen years old. They called it "toxic shock syndrome," but failed to mention that all four of their female patients were of menstruating age, and that three of those women had developed the syndrome during menstrual periods during which they used tampons. One of the young women died, another lost parts of two toes to gangrene after seventeen days in the hospital. This report, published in the British weekly medical journal The Lancet, was largely ignored by the medical profession.

The history of menstruation-associated TSS might be said to begin with a telephone call by Dr. Andrew Dean, the Minnesota State Epidemiologist, to the CDC in January 1980. Dr. Dean reported five cases of an unusual illness in previously healthy women in Minnesota that closely resembled the Toxic Shock Syndrome described by Dr. Todd and his co-workers. Then Dr. Jeffrey P. Davis, State Epidemiologist of Wisconsin, reported seven cases similar to those of Dr. Dean, some of which had been brought to his attention by Dr. Joan Chesney and her husband, both physicians practicing in Madison, Wisconsin. Late in March, a "Disease Alert" by Christian G. Shrock, M.D., of Minneapolis appeared in the Journal of the American Medical Association. Dr. Schrock reported on three seriously ill young women he had treated, each of whom was either menstruating or was just past a menstrual period. One of the three died. Dr. Schrock found herpes simplex virus in two of his three patients and thought that this virus might have caused the disease.

CDC headquarters in Atlanta had been getting a steady stream of reports of TSS. In the *Weekly Report* of May 23, the data were summarized: fifty-two cases had been reported in women since October 1, 1979; physicians in eight states had reported individual cases, while clusters of cases of TSS had been diagnosed in Wisconsin, Illinois, Minnesota, Utah, and Idaho. It was clear that, in the context of menstruation, this was a new disease. In order to begin the epidemiological studies that might yield clues to the origin of the illness, a definition of Toxic Shock Syndrome had to be agreed upon. To ensure that a single disease was being investigated, and not a group of different diseases with some common features, the definition focused on the most striking symptoms of TSS. The official description included fever of 102°F (38.9°C) or higher, a diffuse rash somewhat resembling sunburn, shock— as manifested by low blood pressure (hypotension)—redness of the eyes, inflamed (often fiery red) mucus membranes of the mouth, throat, and vagina, and at least three of the following groups of symptoms that indicated multisystem dysfunction: vomiting or diarrhea (usually voluminous and watery); impaired consciousness (confusion, agitation, somnolence, combativeness, amnesia, etc.); and, as revealed by the appropriate laboratory tests, impaired liver or kidney function, reduction in the blood component called platelets, dysfunction of the heart and lungs, evidence of muscle degeneration, and decreased levels of calcium and phosphorus in the blood serum. The diagnosis of TSS was confirmed when other possible infectious diseases (streptococcal scarlet fever, rash-associated viral infections, Rocky Mountain spotted fever, leptospirosis, and Kawasaki disease, for example) were ruled out, along with drug reactions, by laboratory study.

Many severely ill victims of TSS had all these symptoms and more besides, and because of the abrupt onset of the disease could specify to the hour when it began. Others with milder cases were excluded by this definition, usually because they did not have a blood pressure drop sufficient to meet the criterion for hypotension (a systolic—or maximum—blood pressure of 90 millimeters of mercury; normal is about 120). In contrast to the normal blood pressure of 120/80, women in severe toxic shock measured as low as 50/0.

According to the official description of TSS it has many features in common with Kawasaki disease, a serious illness usually attacking children under five (see chapter 6). Many of the cases of adult "Kawasaki disease" are probably Toxic Shock Syndrome. They are not, however, simply two different forms of the same disease.

By the end of January 1981, the twenty-five members of the CDC Toxic Shock Task Force could give a clear account of the 1980 epidemic. By then, 941 confirmed cases of TSS had been reported, 96 percent of them in menstruating women. Seventy-three cases (nearly 8 percent) were fatal. In the twenty-two months from January 1977 to November 1978 there had been only thirty cases of TSS, three of them not associated with menstruation. Procter and Gamble had test-marketed Rely in small areas of the Midwest since 1974. In August 1978, however, to the accompaniment of a massive promotional campaign that included mailing free samples to millions of homes and free distribution of samples to half a million women college students, Rely was marketed nationally for the first time. Its share of the market rose steadily thereafter.

In August 1978, the number of cases of TSS reported monthly rose above the previous peak of four, first to five, then ten, and finally to seventeen cases a month in July 1979. For the twelve-month period beginning in November 1978, there were 104 cases of TSS, a monthly increase of more than six-fold over the preceding twenty-two months.

That was nothing compared to what was to come. In the single month of August 1980, there were 127 cases of TSS reported: more than there had been in the year ending in November 1978. For all of 1980, the CDC tallied 837 cases of Toxic Shock Syndrome. Of all reported cases, one third occurred in women fifteen to nineteen years old; four cases in five were in women under thirty, presumably because a greater proportion of young women use tampons. Black women, in whom over 100 cases would be expected on a population basis, reported only 7. The reason for this low incidence in blacks is unknown. TSS was reported from every state except Vermont and Alaska, although about one quarter came from Wisconsin and Minnesota. Utah also had a high reported incidence, but the CDC team concluded that this reflected the interest in the disease by local investigators in those states. (A particularly bizzare case occurred in a forty-one-year-old Michigan man who was apparently infected while cleaning out a toilet plugged largely with tampons. Contaminated water spilled over his right knee on which there was an unhealed wound.) Nor was TSS exclusively American. Canada reported seventeen confirmed cases with one fatality (Rely had never been marketed in Canada). Cases have also occurred in Great Britain, Sweden (twenty cases), Germany, Australia, Denmark, France, Iceland, South Africa, The Netherlands, and New Zealand.

Television and the wire services had carried reports on the second CDC *Weekly Report* on TSS in late June, but nothing was said in that report about possible differences in the risk associated with using different brands of tampons. TSS was important to television evening news for approximately two minutes in late June, followed by six weeks of silence while the epidemic exploded. Then, after the third CDC report on TSS on September 19, which mentioned the risk factor associated with Rely, followed in turn by the Procter and Gamble recall and warning campaign, TSS became newsworthy again. *Newsweek* and *Time* picked up the story, and feminist groups began promoting the use of sea sponges as an alternative to tampons.

This was an exceptionally poor idea—the sponges contained fungi, bacteria, and sand, and before long there was a case of TSS in a woman using sponges—but in any event the use of tampons began to drop, ultimately by nearly one third. The trend was accelerated when Rely was withdrawn from the market on September 22. A later report (*Annals of Internal Medicine*, June 1982) found that users of sea sponges during menstruation were more sexually active and more inclined to engage in oral sex than were tampon users generally. More important, they had substantially higher vaginal colonization rates of bacteria (including *Staph. aureus*) than did tampon users. This was not surprising since the sponges, when saturated, were simply rung out, rinsed, and reused within a few hours rather than discarded as were tampons.

The apparent result of the withdrawal of Rely from the market was spectacular. Even though the adverse publicity began late in the month, the number of new cases of TSS reported in September 1980 dropped to 118 (from 127 the month before), at a time when increased awareness might have been expected to increase the number of reported cases. Each subsequent month brought another drop: to sixty-five in October, then sixty-three, finally fifty-five in December. This was still a very high level by the standards of 1977–79, but it suggested that the back of the epidemic had been broken.

By June 1981 only thirty-eight new cases of Toxic Shock Syndrome were reported. This makes the effect of withdrawing Rely even more spectacular. If the reported monthly incidence of TSS in the United States is forty to fifty cases (rather than the one to three previously reported), removing Rely from the market returned the incidence of TSS to normal. For all of 1981, 492 cases of TSS were reported, and tampon use had dropped nearly one third between October 1980 and May 1981.

Of course, it was equally important to know what were *not* risk factors for TSS. In several investigations, a number of factors were shown to be apparently unrelated to the syndrome, among them the method of contraception used (although contraception of any kind reduced the risk of TSS, possibly because of the accompanying sexual activity), frequency of intercourse, including intercourse during menstruation, marital status, number of pregnancies, herpes infection, history of vaginal infection, douching or the use of vaginal deodorant sprays during menstruation, number of sexual partners, intensity and duration of menstrual flow, and the pattern of tampon and napkin use other than the continuous use of tampons during menstruation, which slightly increased the risk of TSS.

On the other hand, several pieces of evidence combined to suggest that Rely was an important contributor to the outbreak. First, there was the eight-fold increased risk factor associated with the use of Rely compared to other brands of tampons, as reported by the CDC team on September 19, 1980. Later, a Utah State Health Department study of twenty-nine TSS victims and ninety-one controls also showed a greatly increased risk (over six-fold) with the use of Rely. There was also the beginning of the TSS epidemic a few months after national marketing of Rely began, and the sharp decline in the number of cases after the product was withdrawn from the market. By mid-1982, four separate studies had shown an increased risk of Toxic Shock Syndrome in women who used Rely.

But none of these bits of evidence proved that Rely caused toxic shock; this could neither be proved nor refuted until the syndrome was better understood. It's also important to note that in a period (April to August 1980) when reported TSS cases rose nearly 300 percent, Rely's share of the market increased less than 5 percent. Reporting of the disease increased in response to publicity about it, and was always more nearly complete in some states than in others.

If Rely did cause toxic shock, as the epidemiological evidence suggested, how did it do so? Women had TSS who used brands of tampons other than Rely, or who didn't use tampons at all, or who weren't menstruating. Men also suffered from toxic shock, although cases of TSS not associated with menstruation amounted to no more than 10 percent of the total in the absence of an epidemic, and far less than that in 1979–80.

One thing seemed relatively clear. TSS resulted from a toxin (or toxins) produced by *Staphylococcus aureus*, the golden staphylococcus, a gram-positive bacterium widely found on the skin and in the nose and throat of humans. More important, it was found in the vaginas of from 2 to 15 percent of women tested for it, although, as we shall see, only a small fraction of them (about one in one hundred) had the strain of *Staph. aureus* that was involved in TSS. Unfortunately, in about two thirds of the cases reported, the organism responsible was not cultured, or the results of such culture were not included with the report. So it remains possible that TSS is a mixed infection (staphylococcal plus streptococcal, for example) in a substantial number of cases.

It was also clear that TSS is a rare disease, affecting not more than 1 menstruating woman in 10,000, although the rate in women under thirty is two or three times higher than in those over thirty. This may be because, from long exposure, older women become increasingly immune to the *Staph. aureus* toxin(s), or because the use of Rely was concentrated in the younger women (eighteen to thirty-four) at whom its advertising campaign was chiefly aimed. The CDC Task Force on TSS estimated that there were approximately 2,000 cases in the United States each year from some 50 million women of menstruating age, of which about one quarter are reported. There are obviously unknown factors that kept the vast majority of women from acquiring the disease. If even 20 percent of women used Rely (and this is lower than some studies indicate), and if the use of Rely inexorably led to Toxic Shock Syndrome, there should have been 10 million cases of TSS rather than a few thousand.

Women who have had an episode of TSS have about a 30 percent chance of a recurrence during subsequent menstrual periods. The current record holder has had five bouts with the disease.

Part of the treatment of TSS is to administer an antimicrobial drug that is not destroyed by penicillin-resistant
organisms. (Most colonies of *Staph. aureus* so far isolated
from TSS victims are resistant to both penicillin and its semi-
synthetic derivative, ampicillin.) This drug administration
does not greatly affect the outcome of the TSS episode being
treated because the organisms are already flourishing and
producing toxins by the time treatment begins, and they can
be removed by removing the tampon and either flushing the
vagina with saline or leaving it to cleanse itself. The drug
treatment does help, however, to kill off the remaining staphylococci so that another TSS episode doesn't arise during a
subsequent period.

Although about 5 percent of TSS episodes were fatal in
1980, death is not due to widespread bacterial infection
throughout the body. *Staph. aureus* was found in the blood
only very rarely, and then usually in women dying of TSS
whose physiological defenses had crumbled in their last hours.
The bacteria were doing their dirty work while growing in
the vagina and making the toxin or toxins that were directly
absorbed from the vaginal walls into the circulation.

One possibility was that the tampons themselves were
contaminated with toxin-producing *Staph. aureus* during
manufacture or packaging. But careful work at the CDC ruled
this out. The bacterium was not present in the unused tampons
of TSS victims nor in the boxes they came in. Packages of all
six major tampon brands were purchased for testing by the
Atlanta team. Although other bacteria were found in the
tampons, *Staph. aureus* was not. The organisms were either
already present in the vaginas of victims of TSS or they
were carried in from the vaginal entrance or the woman's
hands during insertion of the tampon.

The use of tampons causes an increased incidence of
vaginal ulcers. Some investigators also suspected that the
vaginal walls could be injured by inserting the tampons. Although both kinds of injury were possible, there was no evi-

dence for either, based on the examination of living victims of TSS or from autopsies on those dead of the disease, and there was no evidence that frequent changing of tampons raised the incidence, as it should have if insertion injuries were important. A later report (*Annals of Internal Medicine* [A.I.M.], June 1982) described vaginal ulceration in three victims of TSS. Two had used tampons; the other, only napkins.

Nothing seemed to be required beyond the exuberant growth of *Staph. aureus* in the vagina. It wasn't hard to imagine that a fluid-soaked tampon at body temperature was an ideal environment for the growth of bacteria. "Foreign bodies" were known to serve as foci of staphylococcal infection in breast prostheses and in bone infection around staples used to repair fractures. But tampons had been used for over forty years. Why had TSS not been seen earlier?

Possibly a newly evolved strain of *Staph. aureus* was the root of the problem, but despite a rush of new research results in the spring of 1981, this is not clearly established. In February 1981, Drs. Mitchell Cohen and Stanley Falkow of the University of Washington, Seattle, found two small proteins in *Staph. aureus* isolated from women with TSS that did not appear either in laboratory strains of the organism or in colonies of *Staph. aureus* isolated from most women who had not had the disease.[5]

The role of these proteins is uncertain. Less than a quarter of the women who had vaginal *Staph. aureus* but who had not had TSS had the strain of the organism found in TSS victims; it is not clear whether this increases their chances of subsequently contracting TSS.

In April 1981, Dr. Patrick M. Slievert (then at UCLA), and a group of co-workers from the TSS Task Force of CDC reported isolating an exotoxin from *Staph. aureus* cultured from every one of twenty-eight TSS victims but from only one woman in six who had not had TSS.[6] They called this toxin pyrogenic exotoxin C to differentiate it from the dozen other known staphylococcal toxins. This protein toxin is smaller (lower molecular weight) than those isolated by Cohen and

Falkow, but is almost the same size as the toxin whose isolation was reported the following month by Dr. Merlin Bergdoll and his associates at the University of Wisconsin, Madison.[7]

The toxin found by Bergdoll and his associates is called staphylococcal enterotoxin F (SEF). It is also found in at least 94 percent of cultures from TSS victims, but in only 12 percent of cultures from women who have not had TSS. Most of the strains tested by the Wisconsin group also produced staphylococcal enterotoxin A (SEA), which may play a role in Toxic Shock Syndrome.

None of the individual toxins completely reproduces the symptoms of TSS in experimental animals, so it is likely that TSS is the result of the action of more than one toxin (or that humans react differently to the staphylococcal toxin). The toxin of Bergdoll and his co-workers may be the same as that studied by Dr. Slievert and his colleagues.

The SEF of Bergdoll and company has been found in *Staph. aureus* strains isolated as far back as 1947, so the SEF-producing organism is not a new strain, although it may now be much more widely distributed. Another important observation made by the Wisconsin group was that nearly half the women who had suffered a TSS episode and from whom SEF-producing *Staph. aureus* was isolated did not produce antibodies to SEF, although more than three fourths of women who had not had TSS had antibodies to SEF. This may mean that the inability of the TSS victims to produce antibodies to SEF made them susceptible to an initial attack of TSS and to recurrences. It also suggests that SEF-producing staphylococci are widely distributed, so that a large proportion of women have been exposed to them at one time or another and become immune even though, at any given time, only a small fraction of women are hosts to any strain of *Staph. aureus*.

In a recent study of *Staph. aureus* from TSS victims (*A.I.M.*, June 1982), all the organisms isolated produced both pyrogenic exotoxin C and staphylococcal enterotoxin F.

As of April 30, 1982, there were more than two hundred papers in the medical literature on TSS. Since 1970, 1,660 cases of Toxic Shock Syndrome have been reported to the CDC; 88 cases have been fatal (15 in 1981). The disease occurs predominantly in white, non-Hispanic women in their early twenties (65 percent are under twenty-five); at least 88 percent of the cases are associated with menstruation,[8] 99 percent in tampon users. About one third of the victims are fifteen to nineteen years old. The evidence presently available suggests that TSS is a *new* disease.[9] Unfortunately, many important questions about Toxic Shock Syndrome (its true incidence, for example) remain unanswered.

An Institute of Medicine report in June 1982 suggested that women, and particularly adolescents, should avoid high-absorbency tampons. Unfortunately, as pointed out in *Science* on June 18, 1982, that's easier said than done. For example, tampons called "super plus" are usually highly absorbent, but Playtex Super Plus and Playtex Super have the same absorbency. Playtex Regular has the same absorbency as Johnson & Johnson's o.b. Super, and so on. Fluid capacities of tampons may also be changed without public knowledge. Between October 1980 and June 1981, the absorbency of Kotex Super was sharply reduced, and that of Kotex Regular reduced somewhat, but these changes were not publicized.

According to a recent report (*A.I.M.*, June 1982), the highest-absorbency tampons included Playtex Super Plus, Johnson & Johnson's o.b. Super Plus, Tampax Super Plus, and Playtex Super. The intermediate group included Johnson & Johnson's o.b. Super, Playtex Regular, and Kotex Super, while the lowest-absorbency group included Kotex Regular, o.b. Regular, Tampax Super, Tampax Slender, and Tampax Original Regular.

Tampons were first introduced commercially by Tampax, where they were invented in 1937 for use during menstruation. Medicated tampons have been used for contraception since at least 1500 B.C., however; and actresses and professional models had used them during menstruation in the 1800s. For many years, Tampax was the only manufacturer. By 1977, other firms had entered the field so that, by 1980, Tampax had acquired five competitors, and its share of the $700 million tampon market had shrunk. In June 1980, 47 percent of menstruating women used Tampax tampons, but only 21 percent of TSS victims used them. Only 14 percent of women used Rely, but this group accounted for 33 percent of TSS cases. In one study (*A.I.M.*, June 1982) nearly three quarters of TSS victims used Rely, while slightly more than one quarter of matched control subjects did. Under the impact of TSS, however, Tampax's market share has returned to nearly 60 percent.

The original Tampax had been made of pure cotton; they were later changed to rayon or to a rayon-cotton blend. In an effort to increase absorbency, the other manufacturers entering the field began using a variety of synthetic polymers such as polyacrylate, rayon cellulose, polyester foam, and carboxymethylcellulose (CMC). These substances increased tampon absorbency to an almost absurd degree. The average woman loses 50 to 60 cc (about 2 ounces) of menstrual blood over the course of an entire period. Some of the super-absorbent tampons can hold up to 25 cc of fluid. One result is that normal vaginal secretions are absorbed as well, and these fluids are needed to help the vaginal mucosa combat infection. The use of super-absorbent tampons *throughout* a menstrual period seems fairly irrational, and their use generally increases the risk of TSS to some degree.

Rely used CMC as an absorbent and distributed it in the tampon differently from other manufacturers, namely, in a sort of teabag construction with polyester foam. Was there something about CMC or its distribution, or about some other ingredient of Rely, that promoted the growth of toxin-producing *Staph. aureus*? Such an association has been carefully sought in both public health and industrial laboratories; so far nothing has been found and reported in the medical literature.

Ironically, Tampax, a company that makes nothing but sanitary napkins and tampons, had abandoned its time-tested pure cotton tampon to use synthetic fibers as its competition did. Under the impact of the TSS epidemic, Tampax began advertising that "original" Tampax were again available, made only of pure cotton.

Dr. Kathryn Shands, head of the CDC Task Force on TSS, made several important points in television interviews. For example, women who have had TSS should not use tampons for at least several subsequent menstrual cycles to avoid a possible recurrence. Women who have never had the disease will probably not get it, but they should be alert to the appearance of fever, vomiting, diarrhea, sore throat, and so on during their periods. If any of these symptoms appear and the women are using tampons, the tampon should be immediately removed and they should see a physician at once. The onset of shock in TSS can be abrupt and fatal. Prompt and sophisticated medical attention is essential.

Packages of tampons manufactured in Canada now carry a label warning of the risk of Toxic Shock Syndrome, and suggesting ways to reduce it. Some American manufacturers have begun to follow suit with varying degrees of clarity and forthrightness.

Women can reduce the risk of TSS by using tampons intermittently during their periods, switching to napkins at night, for example, and by changing tampons every four to six hours. The risk of TSS is increased by inserting a tampon by hand rather than by using an applicator. Similarly, the use of contraceptive devices that require a woman to insert her fingers into her vagina (diaphragm or IUD) increases the risk of TSS, according to a recent CDC study. It's also important to remember that although TSS usually begins within the first four days of a menstrual period (and most often within the first two), it may occasionally begin as much as a week after the end of menstruation. By early 1982, there had also been several reports of TSS in women who used diaphragms for contraception. In each case, the diaphragm had remained in place for one and a half to three days, sometimes because the woman found herself unable to remove it.

TSS is not a trivial illness. Although its fatality rate had been reduced to about 3 percent by 1982, it can lead to long periods of hospitalization. In one group of thirteen patients, the average stay in the hospital was ten days; the longest was thirty-five. In those victims of TSS whose low blood pressure cannot be promptly restored by administration of fluids (up to 20 liters—5 gallons—in twenty-four hours), drugs must be used to increase blood pressure, otherwise the patient may die. A side effect of such drugs may be loss of circulation in the fingers and toes, ultimately leading to gangrene and amputation. One criterion for a diagnosis of TSS is the dandruff-like loss of skin, usually from the face and trunk, about three days after the beginning of the illness, followed by the loss of skin in sheets from the hands, feet, or both, seven to ten days later.

The disease is frequently accompanied by such severe joint pain that the victims lie motionless in bed, avoiding even small movements. Pain in the muscles is common and may persist long after the acute phase of the illness has passed. Hair, nails, and the voice may be lost, though all are ultimately restored, and there may be a variety of other long-lasting effects that persist for months or years, including difficulty concentrating, memory lapses, and other neurological abnormalities. One sixteen-year-old girl with an I.Q. of 134 (very superior on the Wechsler scale) still had both a reduced ability to concentrate and impaired short-term memory nearly a year after her bout with TSS.

A dramatic addition to the publicity surrounding TSS is what might be called the Houston Toxic Shock Murder Case. One more murder would ordinarily not attract much attention in that homicidal community. But the alleged victim was Joan Robinson Hill, thirty-eight, a beautiful and prominent Houston socialite, daughter of oil millionaire Ashton Robinson, and wife of plastic surgeon Dr. John Hill.

The *dramatis personae* were a strange lot. Joan had been adopted by the fiercely possessive Ash Robinson and his wife under mysterious circumstances; she quickly became the spoiled darling of her new father's eye. Joan began riding at three, won her first horse show ribbon at five, and went on winning at state, national, and world levels. When she went to Stephens College, a women's school in Columbia, Missouri, Ash and his wife leased a suite of rooms near the campus. During this time Joan was offered an MGM screen test, but she turned it down. Then she fell in love and married an Annapolis graduate. When the young couple moved to Pensacola, Florida, so did Ash and his wife, and Ash joined his daughter every morning for coffee. The marriage lasted six months.

Joan's next love was a New Orleans lawyer. They eloped. After a few months, Joan was drawn back to Houston by Ash Robinson's apparent heart attack. Ash offered Joan a new Cadillac, a mink coat, a diamond ring, and—as a clincher—any horse she wanted if she would stay a while. Joan's second marriage collapsed. By her twentieth birthday she had been married and divorced twice.

From 1951 to 1957, Joan played Daisy Buchanan to a gaggle of Gatsbys. Operating from the most garishly vulgar building east of Las Vegas—Houston's Shamrock Hotel—Joan sallied forth to collect blue ribbons in horse shows and almost daily mention in the gossip columns. Spectacularly beautiful, earthy, rich, vivacious—her platinum blond ponytail flying as her Cadillac convertible raced around town—Joan Robinson effortlessly dazzled men and woman alike. John Hill, M.D., was rendered practically speechless.

John, tall, handsome, broad-shouldered, and intensely musical, came from Edcouch, Texas, where his life revolved around the Church of Christ. Then, via Abilene Christian College and Baylor College of Medicine, he arrived at Houston's Texas Medical Center. He had another six or seven years of training before he could begin private practice. It was to be a strange match. The virginal Dr. Hill winced every time Joan said goddam, which was often, and he later told her that he could enjoy sex only if it was illicit. Notwithstanding, in September 1957 they were married. The newlyweds moved into the upper floor of the Robinsons' house. They stayed six years. Then Joan and John Hill bought a magnificent home at 1561 Kirby Drive, in the fashionable River Oaks section of Houston, only a few blocks from Ash Robinson's house at 1029 Kirby. Ash drove over each morning for coffee with his adored daughter, who by now had an equally adored son, Ash Robinson's only grandson.

On Saturday, March 16, 1969, Joan Robinson Hill announced to three of her friends that her twelve-year-old marriage was over. She was consulting a lawyer on Monday. The next day she became ill. Late Tuesday morning her husband took her to a small hospital where he was scheduled to perform surgery (he was also part owner of the hospital). Joan's admission blood pressure was 60/40. She had vomited some and had uncontrollable diarrhea. Her body was swollen, she had a high fever, her blood pressure remained low, and she developed kidney failure. In the early hours of Wednesday morning she screamed for her husband, blood spurted from her mouth, and she was dead.

In clear violation of Texas law, her body was removed from the hospital and embalmed before an autopsy was done.

Ten weeks later, Dr. John Hill remarried.

A grand jury carefully considered the matter of Joan Robinson Hill's death but adjourned without taking action. Convinced that John Hill's precipitous second marriage was the motive for murder, Ash wanted his daughter's body exhumed and examined by Dr. Milton Helpern, medical examiner for the City of New York.

On Saturday, August 16, the body was exhumed. Despite the steel coffin and the embalming fluid, a mask and glove of black mold covered part of Joan's face and one hand, starkly set off by her silver-blond hair and silver nail polish. The nose was crumbling, and wisps of blue-green mold like cobwebs covered the torso. But nothing incriminating was found and the second grand jury investigation came to a halt. Some six weeks later, a third grand jury convened to consider Joan Hill's death; the grand jury indicted John Hill for the murder of his wife. The trial ended in a mistrial. Before a retrial was scheduled, John Hill was murdered in front of his new (third) wife and small son, allegedly by a contract killer.[10]

On the CBS Evening News on Saturday, November 22, 1980, Jim McManus reported from Houston that Dr. Hill's former attorney, Richard "Racehorse" Haynes, now believes that Joan Robinson Hill died of TSS. Many of her symptoms were those of toxic shock. She died within four days of the beginning of her final illness, a time scale consistent with TSS, and she had just completed a menstrual period when she died. Her maid said there had been blood on the towel beneath her employer before Joan was taken to the hospital. Jim McManus interviewed the Houston medical examiner, Dr. Joseph A. Jacimczyk, who disagreed with Haynes's theory, because not all of Mrs. Hill's symptoms fit the picture of Toxic Shock Syndrome. But Dr. Paul Radelat, a pathologist who was present at the second autopsy on Joan, said that the attorney's proposal was entirely reasonable, and Joan's close friend, nurse Dottie Oates, told Jim McManus that Joan habitually used tampons.

So it is possible that Joan Robinson Hill, whose tombstone describes her as "Horsewoman, Wife, and Mother—and a Champion in All," died of entirely natural causes.*

---

* I had written what I believed was a lively and entertaining account of this case. Because of potential legal problems, my account was heavily censored by the publisher's lawyers, leaving what you have just read. Interested readers are referred to Tommy Thompson's book (note 10).

5

Siberian Ulcer
and Yellow Rain

*Each state party to this convention undertakes
never in any circumstances to develop, produce,
stockpile, or otherwise acquire or retain: (1)
microbial or other agents, or toxins whatever
their origin or method of production, of types
and in quantities that have no justification for
prophylactic, protective or other peaceful purposes.*
Signed in Washington, London, and Moscow
on April 10, 1972.[1]

In the beginning it was bad enough. First, an explosion produced a lethal cloud. About a dozen men, scientists and
technicians doing their military reserve duty at Military Compound (or Village) Number 19, sickened and died within
hours some time between April 3 and 6, 1979. Then troops,
camped near the Sverdlovsky State Farm that borders the
military compound and supplies fresh produce to the city,
fell ill as well. In all, there were some 100 deaths in this

group. Worse yet, civilians went on dying at the rate of forty to fifty a day until the middle of the following month. The first to go were the employees—apparently almost the entire shift on duty at the time—of a ceramics plant close to the military compound.

It could have been even more of a disaster. But the god of the babushkas (as Russian grandmothers are called) smiled faintly on the people of Chkalov Borough, and the deadly cloud from the explosion rode the wind southeast out of the pine woods surrounding the military compound, drifting across the sparsely populated peat bogs toward the village of Kashino some eighteen miles away, rather than north over the great city of Sverdlovsk.

Sverdlovsk is the metropolis of the eastern Urals, home to 1.2 million souls, hub of roads, among them the main highway to Moscow 875 miles nearly due west, and an agricultural and manufacturing center. As I pointed out in a previous book,[2] it is also believed to be one of the major facilities in the Soviet Union for the production of biological weapons. The evidence is from satellite photographs that show a characteristic architecture and arrangement. All of the Urals are entirely closed to foreign visitors, with rare exceptions.

The explosion at Military Compound Number 19 sent a dense cloud of anthrax bacilli boiling into the air on the southern border of Sverdlovsk. The anthrax organism, *Bacillus anthracis*, in the spore form in which it is readily produced, is an extremely rugged and highly infectious bacterium that is high on everyone's list of candidates for biological warfare (BW) agents. Anthrax spores are found in soil in most parts of the world, including the United States and the USSR. They are capable of surviving there for decades if not centuries, and cause various forms of the disease in animals and man.

Most commonly, anthrax appears in humans in the skin (cutaneous) form, known in the Soviet Union as "Siberian ulcer" because of the prevalence there of its characteristic black raised eruption. The disease can also be acquired by eating meat from infected animals. Neither cutaneous nor gastric anthrax is trivial, but both are curable with modern antimicrobial drugs, specifically penicillin or the tetracyclines. There is also an effective vaccine for both human and veterinary use. The vaccine contains, at least in the United States, living anthrax spores of an avirulent strain unlikely to cause serious illness.

The most devastating form of the disease, however, is the pulmonary form in which—so the story goes—it struck the citizens of Chkalov Borough. This is the form most useful for biological warfare. In pulmonary anthrax the organisms, most probably as spores, are inhaled into the lungs. In the pneumonic forms of plague and tularemia, for example, the organisms begin multiplying as soon as they find themselves in the rich, moist environment of the deep lung, and infection spreads rapidly across this vast surface (equivalent in area to the outer skin). This leads to the typical light spots on a chest X-ray signifying pneumonia.

In pulmonary anthrax, however, the spores, which are inactive and incapable of multiplying, are captured by the defensive cells of the lung and taken to the lymph nodes in the vicinity of the breastbone (sternum) for disposal. Unfortunately for the victim of pulmonary anthrax, the planned destruction of the spores doesn't work very well. The spores germinate within the defensive cells—inside which they are conveniently safe from antimicrobials—then, in the vegetative form that is capable of growth and multiplication, they spread throughout the body via the lymph and blood circulations. Late in their lives, they produce the anthrax toxin that usually kills their victim. The mortality rate from untreated pulmonary anthrax is about 90 percent. This is not as bad as in untreated pulmonary (pneumonic) plague, but the difference, from the standpoint of biological weapons, may be made up for by the anthrax spore's resistance to sunlight, heat, cold, and disinfectants. Pulmonary anthrax does not spread from person to person as pneumonic plague does. Connoisseurs of biological warfare agents are hard put to choose between plague and anthrax, but anthrax may have a slight edge because of the durability of the spores.

After troops sealed off the area, Soviet authorities almost immediately began immunizing people, particularly the several hundred thousand persons in the industrial section of southern Sverdlovsk. Most people got one injection in mid-April and another two weeks later. It didn't always work. Some of those immunized later died of anthrax. It is unfortunately true that immunization is seldom effective against virulent pulmonary infections like anthrax or plague. The organisms grow happily inside defensive cells and the infection spreads so rapidly that the body has no time to respond with antibody production before fatal poisoning ensues. Nonetheless, the action of the Soviet authorities may have saved many lives.

A sudden cold wave hit the Sverdlovk area shortly after the explosion and this was credited (falsely, I believe) with helping to keep down the casualty rate. As the snow melted, the citizens of Sverdlovsk and its environs were commandeered to clean the streets and the topsoil was removed from an immense area in the inverted Y (nearly 20 miles across the base) between two roads, one of which runs past Military Compound Number 19 to the town of Polevski in the west, and the other to Kashino and Sysert in the east. (The junction of the inverted Y is at the southern edge of Sverdlovsk.) The citizens of Kashino even had the great distinction, in the rural Soviet Union, of having their streets subsequently paved with asphalt to seal in the infection.

Did any of this really happen? It's a wonderful story, but it has a shady and uncertain history. Moreover, the report of thirty to forty deaths a day continuing for most of a month is inconsistent with the usual behavior of pulmonary anthrax, which kills in a few days and is not contagious.

The first word of a biological warfare (BW) accident in the Soviet Union was an account in an obscure Russian language newspaper *Possev* (*Sowing*), published in Frankfort, that appeared in early October 1979. That article, however, referred to an accident in a BW facility in a suburb of Novosibirsk (1,000 miles east of Sverdlovsk) in the spring of 1979. This same story was published by a new British news magazine called *Now!* on October 26, 1979. *Now!* termed the story "Russia's Secret Germ Warfare Disaster," and splashed the title across the magazine's cover. *Now!*'s writer, David Lloyd, said he got the details about an accident in Novosibirsk from a traveler who was present at the time. The article spoke of sealed coffins, bodies covered with brown patches, and so on. Lloyd did admit that the event on which he was reporting could have been a chemical plant accident like the famous incident near Seveso, Italy.

The day following publication of the article in *Now!*, the Hamburg *Bild Zeitung* ran an article about an alleged BW accident in Sverdlovsk in the spring of 1979 in which more than 1,000 persons died. The "Bay Tset" (*BZ*), as it is called throughout Germany, is a tabloid heavy on lurid pictures, bright colors, sex, and gore. It is naturally very popular. In a country of some 60 million, the circulation of *BZ* is 4.7 million.

In early January 1980, *Possev* weighed in with another story in which it admitted that its first story was wrong, and that the whole event described in that story had actually taken place in Sverdlovsk! Meanwhile, the Soviet news agency Tass was having trouble keeping up with the confusing stories in the foreign press. Finally, on February 9, 1980, it claimed that the October story in *BZ* was "from beginning to end a malacious fabrication that has nothing to do with actual facts."[3] The Soviet authorities admitted that there had been deaths from anthrax in Sverdlovsk, but attributed them to the consumption of contaminated meat. Later, they changed their minds and blamed the deaths on an outbreak of foot and mouth disease. Finally, they returned to the contaminated meat story. *BZ*'s reply to Tass was to reprint the second story from *Possev* on February 13, 1980. Then another Russian language newspaper, *Russkaya Mysl* (*Russian Thought*), published in Paris on March 7, 1980, printed a version of the accident of Sverdlovsk presumably acquired from its own sources.

About this time, penetrating remarks were being directed toward the Soviet Union. As U.S. State Department spokesman David Passage said on March 18, 1980, "The disturbing implications that a large number of people [in Sverdlovsk] had been contaminated one year ago by a lethal biological agent raised questions about whether such material was present in quantities inconsistent with the ban on producing, stockpiling, acquiring, or retaining biological agents or toxins."[4]

There was a certain amount of hanky-panky in all this. The Foreign Broadcast Information Service (FBIS), an agency that publishes transcripts of foreign broadcasts and reprints of some articles, had covered the *Bild Zeitung* stories shortly after they first came out. Although they seldom publish anything over two weeks old, the *BZ* articles were reprinted by FBIS on the Friday (March 14) before David Passage's comments. As a senior intelligence officer remarked, "The timing of the reprinting was no accident. . . . [It] was part of a major effort to rev up public opinion about Soviet action in the area of chemical and biological warfare."[5]

Two days after David Passage's remarks, the editor of the Sverdlovsk evening paper *Vecherni Sverdlovsk* wrote that he had published three articles on anthrax in the spring of 1979 as a public service to the agricultural community and not in response to any epidemic. Five days later, the weekly *Literaturnaya Gazeta* attributed the outbreak to foot and mouth disease.[6]

Shortly after *Literaturnaya Gazeta* had put in its two kopecks worth, the British magazine *Nature* published its own article, taken largely from *BZ*, which mentioned that special army nurses wearing protective clothing were being brought in to Sverdlovsk, and that the bodies of those that died were not being returned to their relatives. For good measure, *Nature* also mentioned a rumor of nonfatal infectious hepatitis that had broken out in an area of Czechoslovakia used for training Russian paratroopers when a BW weapon was accidentally discharged. The military hospitals in the area were inundated with patients, according to *Nature*, and the overflow was sent to civilian hospitals in Poprad and Spisska Nova Ves.[7]

On March 27 (two days after the *Nature* article), U.S. intelligence sources said that they had reports from eyewitnesses in Sverdlovsk who provided medical information that eliminated the possibility of a natural outbreak of anthrax. A high-ranking intelligence aide was quoted as saying: "There is no doubt that the Soviets aren't telling the truth."[8]

About a year after the alleged incident, Russian science journalist Mark Popovsky (who emigrated to the United States in 1979 and is now a fellow at the Woodrow Wilson Foundation in Washington) told a reporter from *Science* magazine that he had heard from friends in Sverdlovsk of an explosion yielding a cloud of anthrax bacilli in a compound *north* of the city (the map in the *New York Times* of July 16, 1980, shows Military Compound Number 19 as southwest of Sverdlovsk and Kashino as southeast of the military compound). Popovsky said that he knew definitely of two Soviet BW installations (in Kirov and Sverdlovsk) and had heard of two others (in Kalinin and Novosibirsk). He also mentioned reports of a similar accident in Sverdlovsk the year before, in which tragedy was averted only by an abrupt change in wind direction.[9]

Finally, on July 31, 1980, émigré Soviet scientist Dr. Zhores Medvedev, now working at the National Institute for Medical Research in London, published an article in the British magazine *New Scientist*. Medvedev pointed out the numerous errors in the original story in *Possev* and the version in *Now!*, as well as important mistakes in an article on the subject by Mark Popovsky. Medvedev concluded that the event "was connected either with tainted meat or a laboratory accident. But there are no facts yet to indicate that the production of a bacterial weapon was the cause of the Sverdlovsk epidemic. . . . It is not reasonable to use arguments about the tragedy in Sverdlovsk to revive germ warfare preparations elsewhere."

What really happened at Sverdlovsk? It is conceivable that the "accident" took place in a plant making anthrax vaccine from virulent organisms (as the U.S. plague vaccine is made). If that were the case, the Soviet government could have quashed the rumors by simply saying so and making samples of the vaccine available for analysis. If there had been no accident, however, they might have felt no need to go on talking about something that never happened.

The CIA interpretation of the satellite photographs of Sverdlovsk that they claim show a BW production plant seems plausible. Even if an accident had occurred with a biological warfare agent, however, this is not necessarily a violation of any treaty. The Geneva Convention of 1925 (ratified by the United States in 1975) only prohibits *use* of such agents, while the 1972 Convention prohibits production, development, or stockpiling of "excessive" quantities. Research on BW agents is not prohibited by any agreement, so an accident in a BW research laboratory would not be a treaty violation. Incidently, neither treaty contains provisions for verification because verification of the presence of a small BW facility (of which there could be dozens) is virtually impossible, and some of the seventy-eight industrial microbiological plants in the Soviet Union could be intermittently switched to the production of BW agents.

On Sunday, September 13, 1981, Gen. Alexander Haig, U.S. secretary of state, gave a speech in the Hotel Steigenberger to the Berlin Press Association as a crowd of 30,000 to 50,000 demonstrators paraded in protest and threw rocks at police a few blocks away. The secretary said, "I detect a growing double standard in the West toward applied norms of international behavior." He went on to cite the muted outcry over the Soviet invasion of Afghanistan and the near silence on

the Vietnamese seizure of Kampuchea (Cambodia) as compared with the constant and noisy revilement of the Western
powers, and particularly the United States, over lesser matters:
"For some time now, the international community has been
alarmed by continuing reports that the Soviet Union and its
allies have been using lethal chemical weapons in Laos,
Kampuchea, and Afghanistan. . . . The UN has appointed
an impartial group of medical and technical experts to investigate . . . [but] reports of this unlawful and inhuman activity
have continued."

Then came the punchline: "Moreover, we now have
physical evidence from South East Asia which has been
analyzed and found to contain abnormally high levels of three
potent mycotoxins—poisonous substances not indigenous to
the region and which are highly toxic to man and animals."[10]
Haig promised a fuller discussion at a press conference in
Washington the next day.

That discussion fell to Walter Stoessel, Jr., under secretary of state for political affairs, who told reporters that although the present evidence consisted of one leaf and one
stem sample collected in Cambodia near the Thai border six
months before, previous information from eyewitnesses and
victims extended back over the last five years. He added: "In
June of 1980 we prepared a 125-page compendium of reports
of chemical warfare use as a basis for supplementing the
December, 1980 UN resolution to establish an impartial international commission on [such] use. The compendium was
updated in March, 1981. The levels of mycotoxin found [in
the leaf and stem sample] were twenty times higher than in
any recorded natural outbreak." The results of being sprayed
with such mycotoxins, he explained, were vomiting, multiple
hemorrhages, bloody diarrhea, and severe itching and tingling
of the skin with the formation of small multiple blisters and,
in a matter of hours, death.

The under secretary pointed out that a medical team
appointed by the army Surgeon General had visited Southeast

Asia in the autumn of 1979, interviewed and examined refugees, looked at their medical records, and spoken to eyewitnesses.* Their report was an important part of the State Department compendium. Mr. Stoessel admitted that "certain other agents are being used that we have not yet identified." Symptoms similar to those described were reported from large numbers of people in Cambodia, Laos, and Afghanistan. A State Department fact sheet distributed to reporters at the time of Stoessel's press conference explained that there were fifty years of research effort on mycotoxins in the Soviet Union and that "Preparation [of the toxins] does require . . . large-scale biological fermentation facilities and no such facilities are known to exist in South East Asia."[11]

Time magazine carried a one-column story on the use of mycotoxins in Afghanistan, Laos, and Cambodia in the issue dated the day of Stoessel's press conference, which described the use of mycotoxins by Vietnamese troops in Cambodia.

It was not really a big secret. The Subcommittee on International Security of the House Committee on Foreign Affairs had held hearings on December 12, 1979, on the same subject at which Deputy Assistant Secretary of State Evelyn Colbert had discussed the results of investigations on the use of chemical and biological weapons in Southeast Asia, particularly in Laos. On Thursday, April 24, 1980, at 10:15 A.M. the subcommittee resumed hearings. The use of chemical and biological agents by Soviet or Soviet-sponsored forces in Laos, Cambodia, and Afghanistan was discussed by the under secretary of state for security assistance, science, and technology, Matthew Nimetz; Rear Adm. Thomas B. Davies

---

* The team consisted of Col. Charles W. Lewis, M.D., chief of dermatology at Brooke Army Medical Center, San Antonio; William D. Tigertt, M.D., professor of pathology at the University of Maryland School of Medicine; Dr. Frederick R. Sidell, an expert on nerve gases; and an enlisted man, Sp. 5 Burton Kelley, an associate of Colonel Lewis.

(retired) of the Arms Control and Disarmament Agency; and Prof. Matthew Meselson of the Department of Biochemistry and Molecular Biology of Harvard University.

Mr. Nimetz pointed out that chemical defense battalions accompanied three of the Soviet Army divisions then in Afghanistan, along with the mobile decontamination unit called a TMS-65 that is used for cleaning trucks, tanks, and other large pieces of apparatus contaminated with persistent agents like some of the nerve gases. The TMS-65 consists of a turbojet engine mounted on a truck. All Soviet Army divisions have an attached chemical defense battalion, however, and as Professor Meselson pointed out, the TMS-65 has also been observed spraying insecticides and melting the ice on roads and runways. Since the Soviet troops were unlikely to be under gas attack from the Afghan forces, the appearance of this equipment was consistent with the idea that they might be planning such attacks themselves, but it was certainly not proof.

Tass was not amused by the secretary of state's speech or the sequel. The news agency promptly carried a story denouncing Haig's disclosure as a "big lie . . . libelous and groundless," and pointed out that the United States had used chemical warfare on an immense scale in Vietnam (true, but directed largely against crops and forests), and in Afghanistan (presumably via the anti-Soviet Afghans), as had the U.S.-supported junta in El Salvador.[12] Tear-gas cannisters with U.S. markings (sold to police forces all over the world) had been found in the effects of anti-Soviet forces in Afghanistan. A similar discovery might have been made in El Salvador.*

A colleague and I visited scientists in the State Department and in the Pentagon a few weeks after the Haig speech.

* Soviet authorities (and some U.S. experts) consider that chemical warfare includes biological warfare as well. The lumping together of these two very different kinds of agents under the rubric of "chemical warfare" generates much unnecessary confusion.

The government scientists were still shaking their heads over the secretary's disclosure. In their view, although the evidence of witnesses on the use by the Vietnamese and others in Southeast Asia of "yellow (or red or blue) rain" was substantial, more physical and chemical data should have been accumulated before going public. They feared, though it was never put so bluntly, that the secretary's reputation for loose talk on nuclear weapons demonstrations and the like would serve to weaken the evidence for the use of mycotoxins in Asia.

There is no doubt that the early pronouncement damaged State Department credibility with the scientific community, and it's easy to sympathize with the frustration of scientists faced with the necessity of taking political action on the basis of inadequate data. But, in fact, Secretary Haig may have felt that his hand was forced by the imminent publication of Sterling Seagrave's book *Yellow Rain*,[13] which was on sale in Washington bookstores not long after Haig's Berlin speech.

Yellow Rain is flawed by frequently grotesque writing. More substantively, the author persistently refers to toxins as a third (new) generation of chemical weapons of such potency that they will lift warfare to a new level of horror. Warfare is already as horrible as can be imagined, and toxins, popular with the Borgias, are obviously not new. The mycotoxins on which Seagrave focuses his attention are far from being the superpoisons he makes them out to be, at least on the basis of the limited information now at hand. T-2, the most toxic of the mycotoxins, is about 100 million times less potent than the readily available botulinum toxin, and about one tenth as lethal as the favorite Soviet nerve gas, soman, when either is injected into the abdominal cavity of experimental animals. Although this is an admittedly artificial route of administration, these are the only data available, and such studies have a good record of predicting relative toxicities by other routes of exposure. More recently, however, Dr. Sharon Watson of the Army Surgeon General's office, the army's senior mycotoxin expert, was quoted (*Nature*, March 25,

1982) as saying that recent tests had shown that as little as thirty-five milligrams of tricothecene toxin (about a thousandth of an ounce) could kill half the average American-sized (seventy-kilogram) men exposed to it.

Seagrave also strenuously implies that people poisoned by eating mycotoxins die within hours. In fact, poisoning by mouth is a slow process that may be fatal only after some weeks.[14] Finally, although there are more than forty of what chemists call the tricothecene mycotoxins produced by the various species of the almost ubiquitous fungal genus *Fusarium*, Seagrave refers to all of them as T-2 toxins; only one of them is called T-2.

Despite these and other shortcomings, Seagrave's book is important in emphasizing what has been going on elsewhere in the field of chemical and biological weapons while the United States was sleeping the sleep of the just (and stupid). As Representative Jim Leach (R.-Iowa), a former Foreign Service officer, put it: "Private journalists and university scientists did more to uncover evidence of the use of exotic mycotoxins than did our entire intelligence community."[15] This is true, but it is the result of dismantling, after 1969, that portion of the intelligence community that concerned itself with chemical and biological warfare since these topics were thought to be no longer important.

Seagrave describes interviews with the victims of what appear to have been attacks by mixtures of biological and chemical weapons. The clouds of gas that descended upon them were red or blue (sometimes both) and were often followed by a yellow powder, the putative "yellow rain" of mycotoxin. It's not clear whether the colors were used for psychological effect or represented different experimental mixtures of agents. Alternatively, they could simply have been markers for the pilots of the spray planes to indicate which areas had been sprayed and with what.

The number of people killed in the alleged mycotoxin attacks is also difficult to assess. Seagrave estimates between

5,000 and 20,000. Gen. Vang Pao, former head of the Hmong Army allied with the United States during the Vietnam War, considers that 50,000 persons, many of them children, have died since 1975.[16] The figure given in the State Department report released in late March 1982 is 10,333.

Fungal mycotoxins have been a public health problem in the Soviet Union for decades, and the problem was especially critical in the lean years near the end, and just after, what the Soviet people call the Great Patriotic War (World War II). It is a frequent occurrence in parts of the Soviet Union that unharvested barley, millet, wheat, or other grains are covered by an early snowfall under which they remain until the spring sun melts the snow and dries the fields. Often, in repeated cycles of freezing and thawing, the temperature of the grain under the snow rises enough to encourage growth of the fungus (or mixture of fungi) and production of a battery of mycotoxins. The fungus continues to grow until the temperature reaches as low as 19°F (-7°C); the temperature for maximal toxin production is just a few degrees higher. When the grain can finally be cut, it is contaminated with mycotoxin. In lean years when the peasants can afford to waste nothing, this leads to the illness and death of both farmers and their livestock. In 1944, 10 percent of the population of the town of Orenburg about 400 miles southeast of Sverdlovsk died of what is now believed to be largely poisoning by the T-2 mycotoxin.

Because of this serious problem, research into mycotoxin production has been carried out in several institutes in the Soviet Union. Much of our knowledge of the structure of the various toxins, their biological effects, and their mode of production has come from the excellent work of Soviet scientists. Some of these studies have concerned fermentations designed to produce mycotoxins at maximal yields in order to obtain enough of the material for detailed chemical studies. Such investigations may obviously form the basis for producing mycotoxins for less peaceful purposes. A detailed account of this work was published a decade ago by a former Soviet scientist who worked at the Institute for Epidemiology and Microbiology of the USSR in Moscow and who now lives in Israel.[17] As recently as 1977 a week-long workshop on *Fusarium* toxins was conducted at the Kiev Institute of Microbiology and Virology; and one Soviet facility (Berdsk Chemical Works near Novosibersk) is known to produce *Fusarium.*

It was just six days after Secretary Haig's Berlin speech that a Western diplomat in Bangkok reported some of the 200,000 Vietnamese troops occupying Cambodia had apparently used mycotoxins against a group of Khymer Rouge insurgents. A Western medical worker, no fan of the Khymer Rouge, was present at the hospital in western Cambodia where the victims were taken for treatment and reported that "the victims suffered dizziness and bloody stools." Of several score patients, at least twenty either were killed at the scene of the attack or died after they reached the hospital.[18]

As the autumn of 1981 wore on, more and more samples were submitted to Dr. Chester J. Mirocha, fifty-two, a highly regarded professor of plant pathology at the University of Minnesota, St. Paul. Dr. Mirocha's specialties are mycotoxicology and analytical chemistry. He is ideally equipped to apply advanced techniques to separating and identifying mycotoxins in those samples that contained them and to determine how much of each were present.

The samples to which Secretary Haig referred were very small (about 0.2 grams each, or 1/150th of an ounce). Chester Mirocha was not told what they were or where they came from, and because of the small sample size, he looked only for the toxic components likely to be present in relatively large amounts. He found the three mycotoxins (deoxynivalinol, nivalinol, and T-2) to which the secretary referred.

By Veteran's Day (November 11), 1981, the State Department had what its spokesman, Richard Burt, referred to as "the smoking gun." He told the Senate Foreign Relations Committee about four separate pieces of evidence of the use of mycotoxins in Southeast Asia. Burt, chief of the State Department Bureau for Politico-Military Affairs, went on to testify that "we have concluded that chemical weapons are being used in Afghanistan, but we have no evidence."[19] On June 7, 1982, the *Wall Street Journal* published interviews with Afghan refugees conducted by a United Nations team that strongly suggested that chemical and biological warfare weapons had been used by Soviet forces in that unhappy country.

Richard Burt's four pieces of evidence had again been supplied by Chester Mirocha. Dr. Mirocha has since analyzed a water sample taken from near where the original samples were obtained, as well as two samples of yellow powder scraped from a rock in a Laotian village by a Hmong refugee. All contained one or more of the three principal mycotoxins at high levels. The yellow dust contained T-2 toxin at 150 parts per million, or 150 milligrams per kilogram of powder.

The day after Burt's testimony brought what, if verified, could be the most solid evidence yet of the truth of the "yellow rain" accusations. A special UN team of four experts and their four advisers ended a ten-day inspection tour along the Thai border with Cambodia and Laos, and found "indisputable evidence" that the Vietnamese forces or their proxies had used biological weapons. The team found at least three cannisters bearing Soviet markings and containing yellow powder believed to be the mycotoxin mixture of yellow rain. There has been, however, no further information released concerning this potentially momentous discovery. At the same time attacks similar to those described previously were said to be continuing in the hills of western Laos, according to refugees who had fled the area.[20]

On May 20, 1982, O. Troyanovsky, the Permanent Representative of the USSR to the UN, presented to the Secretary General a critique of the U.S. State Department document of March 12, 1982, that charged Soviet troops and Soviet proxies with the use of chemical and biological agents in Afghanistan and in Southeast Asia. The critique had been prepared by Soviet scientists. For most of the first fifteen pages (of the English translation) the document presented a reasonable rebuttal and made the telling point that, despite the large numbers of alleged attacks, not one piece of hardware used in such attacks had ever been produced (a rocket, shell, or bomb fragment, for example). Unfortunately for the Soviet case, the writers of the document committed the common error of writers everywhere and went on too long; the rebuttal disintegrated into farce. The argument began to unravel when the authors contrasted the incidence of birth defects in North Vietnam (0.4 percent per year) with that in South Vietnam (4.0 percent per year)—where U.S. chemical weapons had been used for defoliation—as evidence that the use of defoliants had produced the higher rate of birth defects in South Vietnam. The problem is, as we shall see in chapter 10, that birth defects in those countries with accurate records run from 2 to 10 percent, depending on what is counted as a birth defect. The figures given for South Vietnam are about the same as those for western Europe, while those for North Vietnam are absurdly low and therefore meaningless.

Not content with that, the Soviet authors launched into what has become known as the "Elephant Grass Theory." This, by means of a complex scenario, blames the appearance of mycotoxins in Southeast Asia on the United States. It involves the American use, first, of herbicides, then of napalm to "sterilize" the soil, followed by the deliberate seeding of the now "sterile" soil with elephant grass, a good host for *Fusarium*. *Fusarium* thus sprang to life in these areas, and *Fusarium* spores were carried far and wide throughout Southeast Asia. This scenario has been greeted with incredulity by Western scientists. *Science* (July 2, 1982) quoted Dr. Paul Nelson of Pennsylvania State University, one of the world's foremost catalogers of *Fusarium*, who described the Soviet theory as "science fiction."

Then, on July 5, 1982, *Chemical Engineering News* published an interview with Dr. H. Bruno Schiefer of the University of Saskatchewan. He had made an investigation in Southeast Asia in February 1982 for the Canadian government, and sent back samples for analysis. Dr. Schiefer was quoted as saying: "Personally, but with reluctance, I would say, yes, toxins are being used" in Southeast Asia. He suggested that a more complex (macrocylic) form of tricothecene toxins may explain the rapid action of the material. This possibility is being investigated (*Nature*, 16 September 1982).

The thirty-one-page report released by the State Department on March 22, 1982, and referred to earlier, summarized the evidence for the use of chemical and biological (toxin) weapons in Laos and Kampuchea (Cambodia), and of chemical weapons in Afghanistan, frequently under direct Soviet supervision. Through the autumn of 1981, according to the State Department report, 226 chemical or biological weapon attacks were made in Laos (causing more than 6,300 deaths), and, through the summer of 1981, forty-seven such attacks were documented in Afghanistan (with over 3,000 deaths). In Afghanistan, extremely rapidly acting lethal agents had sometimes been used; other agents appeared to cause rapid decomposition of the flesh after death.

Bernd de Bruin, a Dutch journalist, photographed a Soviet-built MI-24 helicopter dropping canisters that produced a dirty yellow cloud; five hours later, he photographed the blackened victims in the village that had been attacked. Bruin himself was exposed and suffered swelling and blistering of the skin. A former Afghan MI-8 helicopter pilot reported that Soviet forces had used chemical agents, and that one gas left the skin so soft that a finger can punch through it. Soviet troops in chemical protective gear have been frequently seen in Afghanistan.

The latest attack reported as of May 1982 was on Sokh Sann in southwest Cambodia on March 13, 1982. Attacks in Cambodia are said to be continuing. In the opinion of fifty-one-year-old Dr. Amos Townsend, a crew-cut former air force colonel who is providing medical care to Laotian refugees, "Chemicals of some sort have been frequently used against the Hmong peoples in Laos for the past five years."[21] Townsend took blood samples from nine persons who said that they were victims of an attack with "yellow rain" a month before.[22] These samples were sent to Dr. Mirocha in Minnesota, who, after analyzing the samples, said only that he "suspects HT-2 [a mycotoxin metabolite] might be present," but there was not enough material to be certain.[23]

Puzzles remain about the use of mycotoxins by Soviet-backed forces in Southeast Asia and elsewhere because they do not seem, on the basis of animal experiments, to be particularly effective compared to other readily available compounds. This assumes, however, that rats and humans are alike in their reactions to mycotoxins, and in some ways they are not. For example, although there are massive internal hemorrhages in all species of animals tested (and in humans), only humans (and possibly cats) exhibit the highly characteristic bleeding from mouth, nose, and bowel so typical of mycotoxin poisoning in humans.[24]

There is another even more imposing problem. Presumably, most of the fatalities caused by mycotoxins in Southeast Asia resulted from inhaling mycotoxin, so that the agent was delivered directly to the lungs, although some was taken up through the skin as well. There are no available data on the lethal dose of any mycotoxin delivered to the lungs of humans or any other animal, to say nothing of mixtures of mycotoxins. This gap in our scientific knowledge is being filled by Col. Richard F. Barquist, M.D., and his colleagues at the Army Medical Research Institute of Infectious Diseases, Fort Detrick, Maryland.[25]

What does it all mean? What conclusions can be reasonably drawn from the Sverdlovsk incident and the rapidly accumulating evidence of the use of mycotoxins in Asia, Afghanistan, and perhaps even earlier in Yemen? It's not an easy question to answer.

There are two extreme views about such developments. One view, popular in the U.S. defense establishment, is that the Soviet leadership is rotten to the core and capable of any infamy. The contrary view, expressed recently by demonstrators across western Europe, is that most of the evil in the world is made in the United States and that we export it even more enthusiastically than Coca Cola and Nestles' baby formula. In the view of this latter group the U.S. concerns about Sverdlovsk and mycotoxins are only propaganda. The holders of both extreme views select plausible evidence to support their positions.

If we assume the first view, according to which the Sverdlovsk event was the result of an explosion in a plant producing a BW agent, then the question is why was the Soviet government producing such an agent? It is the nearly universal view in the American defense establishment that biological weapons have little military significance. There is also a strong tendency in the U.S. military toward "mirror-imaging," that is, assuming the Soviet military think the same way they do.[26] If mirror-imaging is correct, then there seems to be little reason for Soviet BW facilities. The mirror-image theory may be wrong, or the Soviet Union could conceivably be producing BW agents for terrorist groups. For this use, unlike for military purposes (except perhaps for counterinsurgency), BW agents have much to recommend them, and there is evidence that terrorist organizations may be thinking along these lines. So far no terrorist organization has chosen to use agents of mass destruction (chemical, biological, or nuclear) although some groups have threatened to do so. There is no guarantee that such threats may not be carried out in the future. In any case, Sverdlovsk remains a mystery that may someday be solved.

The mycotoxin story is quite different. Here there is massive evidence of the use of biological agents, although this evidence is largely anecdotal and not unanimously accepted. A representative of the Mennonite Central Committee traveled extensively in Laos between October 1979 and May 1980 and could find no Hmong who knew of any such attacks.[27] But the growing physical evidence, coupled with the large numbers of witnesses and victims, makes an almost irrefutable case. Why these agents are being used is another question—the benefits seem hardly worth the risks—but that too must await future developments to be answered.

One conclusion that one might draw from the evidence of Sverdlovsk and mycotoxins is that the Soviet military are working diligently to match their already formidable capacity (the largest in the world) to indulge in chemical warfare with an equally diversified biological arsenal.

In 1969 the United States stopped manufacturing chemical weapons, destroyed the stocks of biological weapons on hand, and largely dismantled the research organizations that supported both these areas, along with the intelligence capability to warn us of possible threats. Our ability to defend ourselves against chemical attack is now unsatisfactory; our ability to retaliate in kind is worse. In the area of biological warfare, we are equipped neither to defend ourselves nor to retaliate in kind. I doubt that we will ever want to retaliate in kind, but our defenselessness against both military and particularly terrorist use of biological weapons is disturbing.

One mildly encouraging note in an otherwise grim symphony is that Soviet Foreign Minister Andrei Gromyko in a speech to the UN on July 15, 1982, agreed that a chemical arms treaty should provide for "systematic international on-site inspections" (*Nature*, July 1, 1982). The U.S. government has been pressing for inspection of production, stockpile destruction, and the decommissioning of chemical weapon facilities to which the Soviet government has always replied with a firm "Nyet." It remains to be seen whether Mr. Gromyko's remarks were substantive or rhetorical.

The problems of improved U.S. defense against biological weapons are hindered by the same factors that hinder defense against chemical weapons. These have been described by Amoretta Hoeber (now deputy assistant secretary of the army for research and development) and Dr. Joseph Douglass, Jr. They write of one factor: "While detailed [intelligence] information in its original form should rightly be restricted to a very small community, even the derivative analyses have had an extremely limited audience because of what have been, in the present authors' opinion, unnecessarily constraining levels of classification."[28]

The Hmong tribesman who scraped the yellow dust off the Laotian rock gave the sample to reporters from the magazine *Soldier of Fortune*. Then he is alleged to have said: "Show this to the world. Tell them what is happening to my people. Please ask them to stop."[29]

The last word properly belongs to a Thai officer interviewed in Bangkok by Sterling Seagrave in summer 1982 (*The Wall Street Journal*, September 16, 1982): "What is lost in all this argument is that many people are being systematically murdered with biological poisons for the first time in history." And, after discussing Hitler's extermination of the Jews, he went on: "Now, as then, everybody knows that gassings are taking place, and everybody knows full well who is behind it, so the bickering makes a mockery of human tragedy. It is grotesque, like laughing at Guernica."

6

Slaughter of the Innocents— Two Mysterious Childhood Diseases

> In nearly half the group there was wild delirium,
> with screaming, intense irritability, and violent
> movements, during the period when conscious-
> ness was deteriorating. . . .
>
> R. D. K. Reye, M.D., et al.
> The Lancet, October 12, 1963

On Monday, February 26, 1980, Sherwood Elementary School, a one-story brick building on a low hill just south of Sherwood, Michigan, stood bleak and bereft of its normally boisterous complement of 130 pupils, while the citizens of the community, population 400, sat fearfully in their homes amid the dead, brown fields whose crops of grains and soybeans provide a living for most of the people in the area.

A week before, Mary Dutlinger's eight-year-old son, Michael, a student at Sherwood Elementary, had died of Reye syndrome. Just two months before, Holly Jo Burgett, seven, had died of the disease, and her brother Andrew, six, had been very ill. For a rare malady to strike three children in a

135

small school in such a short time had brought Sherwood and its environs to the edge of panic.

Reye syndrome is named for Dr. R. Douglas K. Reye (pronounced Rye), director of pathology at the Royal Alexandria Hospital for Children in Sydney, Australia, who first described a collection of twenty-one cases in 1963. He had seen the first case a dozen years earlier. Also in 1963, Dr. George M. Johnson, a twenty-six-year-old Epidemic Intelligence Service (EIS) Officer of the Center for Disease Control (CDC) was serving at the state board of health in Raleigh, North Carolina; he reported on five confirmed cases in that state. The sobriquet "Reye's syndrome" was bestowed on the disease complex by Dr. H. Giles of Birmingham, England, two years after Dr. Reye's report.*

Reye syndrome is rare, affecting between one and five out of every 100,000 Americans under the age of eighteen, but its effects can be devastating. There is no cure, fatality rates have ranged up to 88 percent, some survivors have permanent brain damage—sometimes severe enough to require life-long institutional care—and the cause of the disease remains a mystery.

Dr. George Johnson's introduction to the syndrome came at Presbyterian Hospital in Charlotte, North Carolina, the first stop in his investigation of a rash of cases of "encephalitis, unknown cause." "I've never seen anything like it," Dr. Lee Large told the young EIS officer. "This lovely healthy ten-year-old girl was the daughter of a dentist friend of mine. She was well, had the flu, got better, then started to vomit, rapidly proceeding into a coma and death. The post-mortem showed unexpectedly marked brain swelling and a very fatty liver. . . ."[1] As Dr. Johnson was to learn, it was a typical case of Reye syndrome, which is frequently misdiagnosed as encephalitis (inflammation of the brain).

* Reye syndrome is now the preferred term, replacing the earlier Reye's syndrome.

Soon after the death of Mary Dutlinger's son, Sherwood Elementary School closed. Michael Dutlinger died on Friday, February 15. On the Monday and Tuesday following, only twenty-three students attended classes in the five-room school. William Tebbe, the tall, slender superintendent of the local school district, ordered the school closed Thursday and Friday, but planned to reopen it the following Monday. In the interim, however, there was a tempestuous meeting of Sherwood parents, school officials, and public health personnel, the result of which was that Sherwood Elementary School remained closed all the following week. It was a compromise that satisfied no one. Mr. Tebbe could see no reason why the school should remain closed following the two-day suspension of classes, while some parents urged that it should be closed for the rest of the year. As Penny Simmonds, a twenty-two-year-old mother from nearby Union City, said: "People here are sure starting to panic. A lot of people are saying that these health people know more than they're telling us; that maybe Reye's syndrome is contagious, but they don't want to tell us."[2]

In the mass meeting, Mary Dutlinger sounded a similar note: "One doctor says one thing. One doctor says another thing. People don't know what to do." Dr. Ronald Waldeman of the CDC could only reply that "It's very difficult for anyone to have fears allayed by a situation that has frankly stumped the experts."[3]

Sherwood, Michigan, was not alone in its agony, when, following the weekend meeting, the school board voted 4 to 3 to close the school for an additional week, some 12,000 students in six other Michigan school districts had already been excused from classes because of other Reye syndrome outbreaks.

Reye syndrome usually follows a viral infection, most commonly chicken pox or influenza. For the Burgett children of Sherwood, it was chicken pox. Bob Burgett, thirty-one, who describes himself as a former "shade-tree mechanic," is half-owner of a service station in Union City six miles from

Sherwood. The home he shares with his wife, Linda, twenty-nine, sits just off Cherokee Drive, about halfway between Union City and Sherwood, on a high bank above Lake Union. In November 1979, the driveway was lined with stacks of wood for the furnace and Bob's snowmobile stood just beyond the woodpile waiting for more snow. Inside, Holly and Andrew, inured to the spectacular view of the lake from the large windows, compared the number and variety of their pox spots. Holly Jo, who had inherited her mother's slender Nordic beauty, was clearly worried about the spots marring her lovely face.

When the children were nearly over their bout with chicken pox, Bob Burgett went off with a friend on an early morning deer hunt. Holly Jo had slept on a twin bed in the living room. Bob kissed her goodbye and they discussed his hunting trip. At that time, she seemed perfectly normal. Linda was still in bed nursing a bad back that had hospitalized her for ten days just a short time before. It was several hours later that she was awakened by her daughter yelling. When Linda got up, she saw that Holly was staggering about the house, apparently disoriented. Later, the child became wildly active, running frantically from the bedroom to the end of the living room and back again. Then she lapsed into a coma. Linda wanted to take her daughter to their pediatrician, but she was unable to carry her. Finally, Linda called her friend Pat, whose husband Bob had gone hunting with, and Pat and her father came to the house by the lake. While Linda dressed herself and her son, Pat's father carried Holly Jo to the car.

Andrew Burgett was feeling much worse, too. He was unusually pale and quiet and, three times during the twenty-minute drive to the pediatrician in Coldwater, Michigan, Pat's father had to stop the car while Andrew got out to vomit.

After examining Holly in the emergency room of the Coldwater hospital where Linda Burgett worked as an LPN, the Burgett's pediatrician, Dr. Steider, advised that the child be taken at once to the University of Michigan's hospital at Ann Arbor, some seventy-five miles away. By then, Bob Burgett had returned from his hunting trip. He and Linda followed the ambulance to Ann Arbor, while Pat, now responsible for the increasingly ill Andrew, insisted that he be examined immediately.

Five minutes after the Burgetts had arrived at the University hospital, a call came from Coldwater. Andrew was also suspected of having Reye syndrome. Linda's parents set out to drive Andrew to Ann Arbor to join his older sister.

For the Burgetts, it was the beginning of a heartbreaking siege. Linda Burgett stayed with the family of Dr. Pete Saxon, an ear, nose, and throat specialist and an old friend of the family, and spent as much time as possible with Holly Jo. Andrew's stay in Ann Arbor was mercifully brief. After four days in the hospital he had fully recovered and returned home. But for Holly Jo hours turned into days, days into weeks, and still the lovely child lay silently in her hospital bed in a deep coma. Dr. Joseph Baublis, a pioneer in research on the treatment of Reye syndrome and professor of pediatrics at the University of Michigan School of Medicine, told the Burgetts that after Holly had been in a coma for a week or more some degree of brain damage was virtually certain, but there was no way to tell how severe it might be.

Bob and Linda Burgett agonized over whether they wanted Holly Jo to survive if it meant that she would live out her life as a human vegetable. Bob Burgett drove to Ann Arbor whenever he could, and Linda occasionally returned to the house overlooking Lake Union. Meanwhile, the Christmas season approached and the nurses who were caring for the Burgetts' daughter braided fresh holly into her long blond hair.

Then, early on the morning of Friday, December 21, Dr. Saxon called Linda from the hospital: "You better come. Holly's failing fast." Linda Burgett rushed to the hospital. The nurses had bathed Holly, washed her hair as they did every night, and put a clean nightgown on her. The nightgown was one Bob Burgett's mother had made for Holly Jo. Green cloth in the shape of holly was appliquéd to the soft flannel.

Just two evenings earlier, Linda had left the hospital encouraged. She was certain that Holly had responded to her voice for the first time. Linda hoped that the child was finally shaking off the coma that had enveloped her for nearly a month. Now she watched helplessly as her daughter slipped quietly into death. Linda cried, as did Dr. Saxon and the other nurses and doctors who had cared for Holly during that nightmare month. Then it was over.

The ordeal of the town of Sherwood was widely shared elsewhere in Michigan and the United States that year. And the agony that Bob and Linda Burgett suffered was endured by many other parents as well. Holly Jo Burgett's case was exceptional only in that she was hospitalized so long, although it made no difference in the end. Holly Jo's brain had probably been clinically dead after the first few days; the semblance of life and the beating of her heart were maintained only by support systems. Finally, the damage to her brain became so extensive that despite the support systems her heart stopped beating and the acute phase of the Burgetts' ordeal came to an end. Clinicians use the term "respirator brain" to describe the flat electroencephalogram that patients like Holly Burgett exhibit. It is a synonym for brain death.

Although Reye syndrome occurs year-round, cases are concentrated in the first four months of the year, and girls are attacked somewhat more often than boys. When a second child in a family is stricken shortly after the first, the second case—as was true of Andrew Burgett—is nearly always milder. Mortality rates are higher for younger children and, except for those under one year, the incidence rate is several times higher for white children, in Michigan at least, than for black children, and higher in rural children than in urban ones, possibly because of the more ready availability of sophisticated medical care in larger cities. Occasionally, as with Holly and Andrew Burgett, two children in a family will have the disease nearly simultaneously, and a few unlucky children have contracted Reye syndrome a second time. There is even an unconfirmable report of a youngster who has had five bouts with the syndrome in five and a half years. In January 1979, two brothers, aged four and two and a half, and their sixteen-month-old sister were hospitalized in northern Georgia with Reye syndrome at the same time.

In most cases, the disease begins with violent vomiting just as the child is recovering from flu or chicken pox, or from infection with one of some seventeen other viruses. Sometimes there is no discernible preceding illness. Between bouts of vomiting, the child is lethargic although unable to sleep. In the next stage, the youngster may become hyperactive, delirious, and hostile, afterward sinking into a coma characterized by loss of voluntary muscular activity (although the child's pupils still contract in response to light) and deep and rapid breathing (hyperventilation). If the coma deepens, the eyes remain open and the pupils no longer respond to light, while the victim's body becomes characteristically rigid. After this stage comes one of flaccid paralysis and loss of both the ability to breath unaided and the so-called deep tendon reflexes like the familiar knee and ankle jerks. The chances for recovery drop sharply as the child passes through the various stages of coma before medical attention is sought. Commonly, the average time from the beginning of vomiting until death is about forty-eight hours; two thirds of the patients who will die do so within four days of hospitalization.[4] Deepening coma also greatly increases the chance of permanent neurological damage. Nearly one third of the forty-six patients in the 1973–74 epidemic who survived the two deepest stages of coma had some degree of brain damage; one was blind, three had periodic seizures, three were spastic, three had speech problems, and two were "vegetables." Tragically, the younger patients are more likely to suffer residual damage. More than two thirds of the surviving 1973–74 patients under four years old reached the deepest stages of coma, whereas less than one third of the older children did.[5] Proper treatment is designed to stop the progression of the disease into ever-deepening coma. The development of such treatment is the principal advance in the Reye syndrome area in the past ten years.

Unfortunately, the essential treatment is not readily available. It requires a pediatric intensive-care unit manned by a multidisciplinary staff skilled in the heroic measures required by the syndrome in its severest forms. As Dr. Allen M. Glasgow of the ultramodern Children's Hospital National Medical Center in Washington, D.C., puts it: "The treatment of Reye's is one of the most intensive therapies you can imagine. I'd say it's the most intensive in medicine."[6] It's not hard to see why.

Brain damage—which in its most advanced form is the cause of death in Reye syndrome victims—results from the increased accumulation of cerebrospinal fluid inside the skull, leading to extreme pressure on the surface of the brain. The blood vessels supplying the brain run first across its surface before sending branches deep into the interior. The result of the increased pressure is the constriction of these surface vessels, hence the loss of blood, and therefore oxygen, supply to portions of the brain. Without oxygen the brain cells die in a matter of minutes, and the capacity of brain tissue to regenerate, once dead, is somewhere between very limited and nonexistent.

The increase in intracranial pressure continues for two or three days after the victim lapses into a coma. If, during this critical period, the pressure can be successfully relieved and maintained at a normal level, the patient will probably recover and be free of serious aftereffects. As Dr. Peggy Hansen, professor of neurology and pediatrics at Albany Medical College, New York, explains: "The aim is maintaining the patient for two or three days. Within that time the disease will have proved fatal or will have cured itself."[7] If attempts to relieve the intracranial pressure fail, the patient will die or suffer permanent brain damage leading to mental retardation, deafness, blindness, or some combination of all three.

When Reye syndrome was first recognized in the early 1960s the importance of reducing intracranial pressure was not appreciated, and up to 88 percent of the children with the syndrome died, while many of the survivors had permanent brain damage sometimes severe enough to warrant lifelong institutional care. Once physicians become more aware of the disease, ways to measure and control intracranial pressure were tried. Now a neurosurgeon may carefully implant a sensor either in the subarachnoid space between two of the three membranes (meninges) covering the brain, or into the fluid-filled cavities (ventricles) of the brain itself. It is not a procedure for the faint-hearted or inexpert. With the intraventricular catheter, small amounts of cerebrospinal fluid may also be withdrawn directly from the brain to help lower the pressure.

A urinary catheter is inserted into the patient. Tubes in the veins and arteries monitor blood gases and pressure. Substances that neutralize stomach acid are passed by tube into the stomach to prevent ulcer formation since acid continues to be secreted, even though the child is receiving all nourishment intravenously. A variety of other treatments designed to decrease overall metabolic rate and hence intracranial pressure may also be administered. The child's rectal temperature may be reduced to as much as 10 degrees (F°) below normal by lying on a refrigerated mattress, and total muscular paralysis can be induced with drugs like curare. This requires that the patient be put on a respirator. Blood transfusions may also be carried out until nearly all of the child's blood has been replaced. This dilutes out toxic factors that may play a role in the progression of the disease, helps control blood clotting problems that usually develop, and reduces blood ammonia, which can reach very high levels in some victims of the disease. Antibiotics and repeated enemas both act to lower blood ammonia levels by decreasing the bacterial decomposition of amino acids in the bowel.

Since the child must be fed intravenously, the physician can add osmotic diuretics to the intravenous fluid, thus drawing water from the cerebrospinal fluid and reducing its volume and the intracranial pressure. In a further attempt to reduce intracranial fluid volume, physicians usually only give less than half the amount of intravenous fluid that would be given to a child who needed intravenous feeding but had another ailment. Mechanical hyperventilation with a respirator also helps to control intracranial pressure.

In extreme cases the child may be given so heavy a dose of barbiturates, commonly pentabarbital, that a coma would result from the drug level alone if the patient were not already comatose. In this condition, the electroencephalogram is nearly flat and the pupils no longer dilate. The victim's eyelids must be taped shut and the eyes flushed periodically with artificial tears to prevent corneal ulcers. The barbiturate coma effectively reduces intracranial pressure but, in some cases, the child never regains consciousness even after the pressure on the brain is reduced and barbiturate administration stopped. At best, it may take a week after the end of sedation for the child to come out of barbiturate coma.

Finally, if all attempts to control intracranial pressure by other means fail, a neurosurgeon is again called in. This time the surgeon removes flaps of bone from the forehead to give the brain more space in which to expand. The flaps of bone are frozen in sterile packages and, if the child recovers, he or she wears a hockey helmet for three or four months until it is safe for the neurosurgeon to replace the bone.

Between 1975 and 1980, five patients of Dr. Allen Glasgow and his colleagues in Washington, D.C., have undergone such surgical decompression of the brain (craniectomy). Of the five, two died, two had severe and permanent brain damage, and one is doing well a year later.[8] Without craniectomy all would probably have died. If the procedure had been performed in an earlier stage, perhaps all the children would have recovered completely.

All these treatments are controversial; various medical teams choose combinations of the possible therapies. In recent years, the ghastly mortality rate of Reye syndrome has dropped steadily. This is in part because of increasingly effective treatment to control intracranial pressure during the critical two or three days. It is also partly because of the fact that, with the increasing publicity given to Reye syndrome, milder cases with an excellent chance of complete recovery are being diagnosed. Of the forty-two cases studied by Allen Glasgow and his associates, thirteen had "benign" disease. Only three of this group required more than minimal treatment to prevent progression of their illness. Andrew Burgett's illness would have been classified by Dr. Glasgow as benign.

Another thirteen patients were considered "treatable" by the Washington, D.C., team. Of these, two suffered severe mental retardation; the others made a normal recovery. The remaining twelve cases were classified as having "malignant" Reye syndrome because their disease progressed to late stages despite treatment. Of this group, seven died, two were retarded, and three made a normal recovery. The oldest victim, whose disease was only diagnosed at autopsy, was a twenty-six-year-old woman. Three other patients died so soon after admission to the hospital that their disease could not be classified. Even among those patients who made a "normal" recovery, some had subtle personality changes and loss of small muscle coordination that were impossible to measure accurately since the children had not been tested before they became ill. Some of these subtle effects will probably disappear in time.

In the April 1982 issue of the *Journal of Pediatrics*, Dr. Timothy Frewen and his colleagues at the Children's Hospital of Philadelphia reported on their efforts to forestall a rise in intracranial pressure by prophylactic pentabarbital coma and hypothermia (reduced body temperature). Superficially, the results were encouraging. Nearly half again as many patients made a good recovery under this regime as when treatment was postponed until intracranial pressure was already elevated, and the fatality rate was reduced from 50 to 35 percent. Less careful workers might have trumpeted these results from the rooftops, but one of the most encouraging trends of modern clinical research is that most investigators now have, and most journal editors now demand, a more sophisticated command of statistics than was formerly the case. Dr. Frewen and his colleagues examined their data carefully and concluded that their results had no statistical significance. Only a much larger and carefully designed study can show whether this prophylactic treatment is beneficial.

The increasing awareness of Reye syndrome has come about through a combination of factors. In late 1973, the Federal Center for Disease Control began national surveillance to monitor the occurrence of Reye syndrome and to publicize its findings in the *Mortality and Morbidity Weekly Report* that was sent free to interested physicians and others concerned with public health matters. This led to an increasing number of research papers appearing in medical journals on the incidence, detection, and treatment of the disease. A very important contribution to public awareness has also been made by the interest groups begun by parents, invariably those who have themselves lost a child to the disease, which publicize Reye syndrome and push for increased research aimed at preventing, or at least effectively diagnosing, the disease complex.

The oldest and largest of these organizations is the National Reye's Syndrome Foundation of Bryan, Ohio, whose president is John Freudenberger. John's wife, Terri, is secretary of the organization, which has well over 5,000 members in 28 states. An imposing collection of scientists and physicians serve as consultants and members of the Foundation's Scientific Advisory Board.

In the late summer of 1974, Tiffini Freudenberger, five, began vomiting. The next morning her mother noticed that Tiffini's eyes were wandering and she appeared disoriented. The Freudenberger's pediatrician, sight unseen, prescribed a drug to control the vomiting. The drug failed and Tiffini grew steadily more lethargic. Finally, the pediatrician agreed to see the child and immediately had her hospitalized. Tiffini was soon diagnosed as a case of Reye syndrome and transferred to a Columbus, Ohio, hospital. She died on Sunday morning, less than three days after her illness began.

It is almost a four-hour drive from Columbus to Bryan, Ohio, and the Freudenbergers had plenty of time to think on their somber journey home after Tiffini's death. Like most parents in such a situation, they were angry and resentful. As John Freudenberger said later: "We were mad because Reye's syndrome had killed Tiffini and we didn't know anything about Reye's."[9] In August of that year they started the Foundation, which had eighty chapters in twenty-eight states as of March 1981. The Foundation runs scientific meetings devoted to Reye syndrome and publishes the proceedings in the *Journal of the National Reye's Syndrome Foundation*, two issues of which appeared in 1980. The Foundation has held six annual meetings, including, in 1981, one in Vail, Colorado. It supports some research from its own funds, and vigorously lobbies for additional support of research by the National Institutes of Health and the Centers for Disease Control.

There are at least two other foundations concerned with Reye syndrome. Some two years after the formation of the Freudenbergers' organization, John Dieckman founded another National Reye's Syndrome Foundation in Michigan. In 1980, a third group splintered off from the Michigan National Reye's Syndrome Foundation to form the American Reye's Association, based in Denver, Colorado.

In November 1976, John Dieckman's eleven-year-old son contracted the disease and passed into a deep coma. He recovered and returned to his home in upper Michigan in December. On his first evening at home he got up in the middle of the night. He explained to his alarmed parents that he was all right and had just gotten up to go to the bathroom. Then he took a few steps, suffered a massive heart attack, and died. In an effort to focus additional attention on the disease that had killed his son, John Dieckman formed the second National Reye's Syndrome Foundation. This organization now has some 3,000 members in 35 states.

The current president of the Foundation's Michigan region is a woman named Dana Allen, much of whose considerable energy goes into speaking to various groups about the syndrome. Her involvement with the malady began when her six-year-old daughter, Chrissie Lee, began vomiting toward the end of a bout with chicken pox on Thursday afternoon, March 22, 1979. The Allens' pediatrician was reluctant to see Chrissie because the child was still in the infectious stage of chicken pox. Chrissie went on vomiting from four o'clock Thursday afternoon until about midnight Friday night. Dana had called the pediatrician's office repeatedly but was told that as long as there were no changes in her daughter's personality the doctor did not want to see her. Dana Allen was told in almost as many words that she was overreacting to her daughter's illness.

Saturday morning, Art Allen went in to check on his daughter and was unable to wake her. Alarmed, he insisted that they take Chrissie to the pediatrician's office. Dana had brought her there once before during her daughter's illness, at lunch hour when there were no other patients around, but had been sent home with comforting words. Now it was too late.

Chrissie was thoroughly dehydrated from her long siege of vomiting. While she was lying on the examining table in the pediatrician's office, Dana tried to give her daughter a drink of water. Chrissie rose to her hands and knees, her eyes glazed and her normally angelic face contorted with rage. She screamed at her mother and tried to bite her. As Dana describes it, "She was like a wolf." Dana went rigid with shock. It was hours later before she could open her clenched fists. The Allens' pediatrician wanted Chrissie taken to the hospital immediately by ambulance. Dana would not leave her daughter, but the doctor would not permit her to ride in the ambulance. Everyone became very angry. The impasse was resolved when Art Allen, 6 foot 4 inches tall and massively built, threatened the pediatrician with an untherapeutic laying on of hands if his wife could not accompany Chrissie to the hospital in the ambulance.

When the ambulance reached Children's Hospital, Chrissie was taken to pediatric intensive care while Art and Dana went to the admitting office. The clerk had to put a pencil into Dana's clenched fist so that she could sign the admitting papers. For forty-six hours the Allens stayed at Children's Hospital. Monday afternoon at 4:00 P.M., almost exactly four days from the time she began vomiting, Chrissie Lee Allen died.

It was a terrible shock, especially for Art, who had been convinced that everything was going to be all right. As he said, "You do everything you can to raise your kids right. You feed 'em well and make sure they get all the shots they're supposed to have—and then something like this." Eighteen months after his daughter's death, the big man's voice still broke when he talked of it.

The Allens asked for cash donations in lieu of flowers at Chrissie's funeral. They both wanted to do something to ease their feelings of utter helplessness and guilt that there might have been some action they could have taken to save their daughter's life. Chrissie was attended in her last illness by a Filipino doctor who is a recognized expert in the diagnosis and treatment of Reye syndrome. The Allens took him the $1,700 they had collected and pleaded with him to use it for research on the disease that killed their daughter. He refused it, saying, "There's nothing you can do. Go home and cry."

They did. But they soon realized that there *was* something they could do, and they began to talk to other parents who had lost children to Reye syndrome. They weren't hard to find. Michigan had ninety cases and seventeen deaths in 1978–79, and eighty-three cases and five deaths the following year. In this way, the Allens learned of John Dieckman's Foundation.

Reye syndrome is a reportable disease in only sixteen states, but, since 1973, the CDC has been urging state health departments to collect information on cases of the disease within their states and to transmit this information to Atlanta. In the seventeen years from the discovery of the disease to 1980, over 1,500 cases have been reported from some forty states. The statistics remain, however, basically unreliable because reporting by individual physicians is mostly voluntary, the disease is frequently diagnosed under the catchall term "viral encephalopathy," and fatal cases are much more likely to be reported than the very mild infections at the other end of the syndrome's spectrum. A later calculation made at the National Center for Health Statistics (a part of the National Institutes of Health) estimated that there were 2,650 deaths from Reye syndrome in 1977. The mortality rate for that year was estimated at 42 percent by the CDC; therefore there were between seven and eight thousand cases of the syndrome in that year. The CDC currently estimates that there are 600 to 1,200 cases of Reye syndrome in the United States each year.

The number of Reye syndrome cases rises whenever there is an epidemic of influenza A or, particularly, of influenza B, as in 1973–74, 1976–77, and 1979–80. In those seasons the influenza-epidemic curves and the curves for Reye syndrome are virtually superimposable. Cases of Reye syndrome related to chicken pox occur primarily in the first half of the year, so they overlap the influenza-related cases but extend further into the spring. There were 221 cases reported from December 1, 1980, through April 30, 1981, compared with 304 the previous year, 93 in 1978, 250 in 1977, and 262 in 1974. The corresponding mortality rates have been dropping steadily, from 88 percent in the late 1960s to 41 percent in 1974, 22 percent in 1980, and 28 percent in 1981. In 1977, 11 percent of the survivors of Reye syndrome had neurological damage of varying degrees. Later studies suggest a several-fold higher (up to 61 percent) incidence of neurological disorders.

There is independent evidence that the improvement in mortality rates is not solely due to more reporting of mild cases, since the mortality rates have dropped in recent years even among children in comparable stages of coma. For example, in 1974 half the children hospitalized at an intermediate stage of the syndrome's progression died, while four years later, the mortality for the same group had dropped to one third.

Reye syndrome has been reported from at least twenty-one countries of the Americas, Europe, Asia, Africa, Australia, and New Zealand. The February 20, 1982, issue of the *South African Medical Journal* describes twenty-one cases seen in three Johannesburg hospitals over a five-year period. Of these, eighteen patients died; the three survivors all had severe brain damage. Reye syndrome, however, is considered a public health problem only in Thailand and the United States. In Thailand, the disease is concentrated in Udorn Province in the northeast part of the country. This variant of Reye syndrome (called Udorn encephalopathy) causes a mortality rate of about 70 percent.

There are three principal theories concerning the cause, or causes, of Reye syndrome in the United States, and it must be kept in mind that the disease may be caused by different agents in different people. The syndrome may also be multifactorial, that is, it may be caused by the combination of several factors, each of which must be present to produce the disease.

One possibility is that Reye syndrome is the result of infection by a second unknown virus, following the preliminary infection with, for example, influenza or chicken pox virus. No such unusual virus has been found so far, though children with the syndrome are often infected by more than one virus. A second theory suggests that susceptibility to Reye syndrome is a consequence of a particular genetic makeup. The third explanation is that the syndrome is the result of exposure to some toxic substance in the environment that weakens the victims' ability to defend themselves against the viral infection, which then progresses to the dramatic neurological complications so typical of Reye syndrome. Alternatively, a preceding viral infection may simply weaken the body so an environmental toxin can make its influence felt.

It is likely that Reye syndrome is a condition that basically affects the subcellular particles called mitochondria, the energy-producing organelles of the cell. The mitochondria of a victim's liver are swollen and disorganized, and the liver cells have lost most of their normal energy store (the carbohydrate polymer called glycogen) and replaced it with vast amounts of fat. The brain mitochondria of Reye syndrome victims are similarly affected though not so dramatically. The damaged liver releases intracellular enzymes such as the transaminases into the blood and can no longer effectively utilize the ammonia formed in amino acid metabolism. Thus ammonia, too, appears in the blood in greatly elevated quantities. The fatty liver, which is so striking in Reye syndrome, is also caused by a number of liver toxins such as chloroform, benzene, and excessive consumption of alcohol. But the brain disease (encephalopathy) that is so important and dangerous a feature of Reye syndrome does not appear in the other conditions that give rise to fatty liver.

There is evidence that the energy metabolism of Reye syndrome victims is genetically deranged, but how these derangements lead to the syndrome, or why the occurrence of the disease in more than one child in a family is rare, remains unexplained. The latter fact is also difficult to reconcile with the idea of an environmental toxin since all the children in one family would be exposed to any toxin in their environment. Moreover, a sophisticated search for toxic substances in the blood or tissues of victims of Reye syndrome has conspicuously failed.

Dr. Larry Davis, a neurologist at the University of New Mexico School of Medicine, and his colleague Dr. Linda Cole are studying an animal model for Reye syndrome in which high levels of influenza virus are injected intravenously into mice. Even though the virus does not multiply in either brain or liver, the animals develop coma, accumulate fat in the liver, suffer a vast increase in liver enzymes in the blood, tend toward seizures, and finally die. These results are presumably due to a toxin associated with the flu virus; further study may provide a clue to understanding the symptoms characteristic of the human disease.

Another approach has been to examine the serum of victims of the syndrome for substances capable of producing some of the symptoms of Reye syndrome in experimental animals. Dr. Doris Trauner of the Division of Neurology at the University of California Medical Center, San Diego, found that slow administration to rabbits of an eight-carbon fatty acid (octanoate) that is high in the serum from Reye syndrome patients causes a rise in intracranial pressure, coma, and then death, with changes in some brain components similar to those in the brains of human victims. Dr. June Aprille of the Biology Department of Tufts University in Medford, Massachusetts, found that Reye syndrome serum causes very unusual changes in rat-liver mitochondria. Her studies show that the responsible factor in the serum increases to a high level and remains there in those patients who ultimately die of Reye syndrome, but that the level declines in the serum of those patients who recover. This factor is now known to be uric acid, a product, like the transaminases, of the breakdown of cellular constituents.

The June 11, 1982, issue of the *Morbidity and Mortality Weekly* reported the Surgeon General's recommendation that aspirin not be given to children suffering from influenza and chicken pox. The same warning was repeated in the June issue of *Pediatrics* and was given wide coverage in the news media. Also on June 11, the *Journal of the American Medical Association* carried an article by Dr. Ronald Waldeman of CDC and his colleagues from CDC and the Michigan Department of Health on the epidemiological basis of the recommendation. They concluded: "Should there be a group of children who are susceptible to the hepatic [liver] effects of both viral infection and salicylate [aspirin] ingestion, clinical illness might develop when the two occurred simultaneously." The authors point out that this idea is totally speculative, but their data clearly show association between aspirin use and the development of Reye syndrome that is not shown when acetaminophen products (Tylenol, for example) are used in place of aspirin.

Much less widely publicized was the report of Drs. John Wilson and Don Brown of the Louisiana State University Medical Center—Shreveport, which followed the report of the Committee of Infectious Disease in the June 1982 issue of *Pediatrics*. They concluded that cases of Reye syndrome were improperly matched with controls for the severity of the illness preceding Reye syndrome. Although temperature was considered in matching cases and controls, dehydration and gastrointestinal disturbance were not. In the opinion of Wilson and Brown, this mismatching of cases and controls invalidates the conclusion about the relation between aspirin administration and Reye syndrome.

So, in laboratories, hospitals, and homes around the world, the struggle against Reye syndrome goes on. Sherwood Elementary School, where our story began, again stands lonely and silent on its little hill, victim this time not of disease but of budgetary problems and shrinking enrollments. In the spring of 1980, the schoolchildren planted a tree beside the entrance and put up a plaque on the wall above it with a picture of a verdant, spreading tree and the legend: "In Loving Memory of Holly Jo Burgett and Michael Dutlinger. . . ." Like the two children and the school, the little tree—once so full of promise—is now dead.

Rochester, New York, Christmas Eve, 1979: A nine-year-old girl is even more flushed with excitement than is usual on such a grand occasion. But then, instead of opening her presents, she is hospitalized with an extremely high fever. A week later, the fever is gone but she is left with a weakened spot (an aneurism) in one of her coronary arteries that may, at best, leave her susceptible to premature heart disease (arteriosclerosis and myocardial infarction), and, at worst, cause a fatal hemmorhage a month or two after her illness. In a three-month period beginning in October 1979 twenty-two other Rochester children suffered from the same ailment.

Boston, March, 1980: A two-year-old boy has a high fever (103° F), red eyes, a sore throat. The pediatrician first prescribes an antibiotic for "a bug that's going around." A few days later, the child has a rash of flat red spots on his arms and legs. His doctor stops the antimicrobial drug because he suspects the little boy is allergic to it. The rash continues to spread, the fever remains high, and lymph nodes in the child's neck begin to swell.

The baffled pediatrician describes the case to a consultant. He points out that his patient clearly does not have German measles (rubella); the disease isn't chicken pox because there is no fluid in the red spots of the rash; it isn't measles because there is no history of exposure and the boy has been immunized against it. Rocky Mountain spotted fever, a disease now rare in the Rockies but common in the East, is out because the spots don't look like the tiny bleeding spots of that disease and there are no tick bites on the boy's body. The hospital lab has not cultured streptococcus, so it can't be scarlet fever, neither were there staphylococci nor any other such organisms, so it probably isn't a bacterial infection. The child's lips, palms, and the soles of his feet are fiery red, as is the lining of his mouth. His hands and feet are swollen and he has a "strawberry tongue"—that is, the papillae on the surface of his tongue are swollen and red.

Late in the second week of the boy's mysterious illness his fever continues unabated and the skin begins to peel away from his fingers and toes starting around the nails. At this last bit of information the pediatric consultant suddenly has the look of one who has seen the light. . . .

Two years before Dr. R. D. K. Reye published his epochal paper on the disease that now bears his name—and some 5,000 miles north of Sydney—Dr. Tomisaku Kawasaki, a thirty-six-year-old Tokyo pediatrician, puzzled over the fact that several of his patients at the Japan Red Cross medical center had the symptoms of scarlet fever but did not respond to penicillin. Over the next six years he became convinced that he had discovered a new disease that primarily struck children under five. By then, he had seen fifty cases. Dr. Kawasaki published his findings in the Japanese *Journal of Allergy* in 1967, and again, with three colleagues, in *Pediatrics* in 1974. In the later report the four doctors called the disease mucocutaneous lymph node syndrome. For obvious reasons, it is most commonly referred to as Kawasaki disease.

Two thirds or more of the victims of Kawasaki disease have cardiac abnormalities during the acute phase of their illness and up to one third develop potentially fatal aneurisms in the arteries supplying the heart, the kidneys, or other parts of the body. Large doses of aspirin are often prescribed by physicians treating the disease, and this may reduce the incidence of coronary aneurisms. For children with heart problems resulting from Kawasaki disease, the aspirin treatment may be continued for up to two years. One-year-old victims have suffered fatal heart attacks subsequently, and sudden death may occur up to eight years afterward.[10] Most cases occur in children under four, most rapidly fatal cases in children under two, and boys are affected somewhat more often than girls. Kawasaki syndrome in children over ten is rare. Only about 2 percent (one in fifty) of the Japanese survivors of Kawasaki disease die of heart attacks, ruptured aneurisms, or cardiac arrythmias that cause the heart to beat so erratically that adequate blood supply to vital organs is lost.

Like Reye syndrome, the cause of Kawasaki disease is unknown, although it is endemic in Japan, where more than 24,000 cases have been reported. Some of the symptoms, and the occurrence of epidemics, strongly suggests that the cause of Kawasaki syndrome is an infectious agent.[11] Treatment is supportive rather than curative. In each case the disease runs its course unimpeded by the efforts of the physician, who can only hope to limit the damage done.

Kawasaki disease has also been reported in South Africa, Canada, Greece, West Germany, Belgium, Australia, Holland, and Italy. The first reported case of Kawasaki disease in the United States occurred in Hawaii in 1971; since 1976, about 100 cases have been reported each year. As with Reye syndrome, this is the tip of the iceberg. There is no requirement for state health departments to report Kawasaki disease and, as Dr. David Bell of the CDC explains, "Even now a lot of doctors in this country have never heard of the disease."[12] The natural result is misdiagnosis, but the beleaguered pediatrician can hardly be blamed. A major criterion for the diagnosis of Kawasaki disease is that it isn't anything else. The list of possibilities to be eliminated, besides those already mentioned, includes drug reactions, meningococcemia or leptospirosis (infection with the gram-negative meningococcus or with the spirochete bacteria known as leptospira), a number of viral diseases, juvenile rheumatoid arthritis, and several others. Eliminating all possibilities other than Kawasaki disease is a tedious and exacting process—frustrating to the physician, costly to the patient.

Outbreaks of Kawasaki disease in clusters improve the chance that cases subsequent to the first recognized case will be promptly diagnosed. The first documented epidemic outside Japan occurred on the island of Oahu, Hawaii, between February and August 1978 (*Journal of Pediatrics*, April 1982), and involved thirty-three children. The victims were predominantly Japanese whose families had lived in Hawaii for three or four generations; the island population at the time was 25 percent Japanese and 30 percent Caucasian. The affected children were predominantly from high income families (nearly half had incomes over $30,000 a year), and nearly half the children had had a respiratory illness in the preceding month. An exhaustive epidemiological study and a search for the causative agent failed to reveal the source of the outbreak.

In Boston in the spring of 1980, there were five cases of Kawasaki disease, and fifty-two others were reported elsewhere in eastern and central Massachusetts at the same time (April–

June), involving some eight counties and children ranging in age from four months to fourteen years.[13] There was no known contact among any of the children. Kawasaki disease, like Reye syndrome, is not infectious from person to person, and some children have had Kawasaki disease more than once, yet no two people in the same family have ever been reported to have it.

Although, as with Reye syndrome, most cases of Kawasaki disease occur in individuals scattered across the country, Massachusetts is the sixth U.S. region to suffer an epidemic of this mysterious disease. The others are Rochester, New York; Hawaii; Richmond, Virginia; New York City (forty cases); and Los Angeles County (twenty cases). A twenty-six-year-old woman (a pathologist) in La Jolla, California, and a twenty-eight-year-old man in Cedar Rapids, Iowa, both contracted Kawasaki disease. The physician, naturally enough, treated herself for the first four days of her illness but then, acutely ill, she put herself under the care of a colleague and was immediately hospitalized. The male victim spent three weeks in an Iowa hospital. Both recovered.

Despite an intensive continuing investigation of the Massachusetts epidemic, the largest in the United States so far, there are still no clear-cut clues as to the origins of Kawasaki disease although a team from Walter Reed Army Institute of Research, the University of Illinois, and Miyaski Medical School in Japan have preliminary results that may link Kawasaki disease and a widespread rickettsial disease of dogs.[14]

Children with Reye syndrome have taken more aspirin (acetylsalicylic acid) and have higher blood salicylate levels than do children with other fever-producing diseases; the salicylate level correlates with the severity of symptoms of the Reye syndrome victims, and salicylate is a mitochondrial toxin. Damage to liver and brain mitochondria is characteristic of Reye syndrome. Although aspirin administration to children potentially suffering from this disease is both unnecessary and undesirable it is still far from clear, however, that aspirin "causes" Reye syndrome.[15]

We may only hope that future research will quickly discover the cause or causes of both Reye syndrome and Kawasaki disease* and stop the loss of lives that results from these two mysterious killers of children.

---

* In a recent outbreak of twenty-three cases of Kawasaki disease in the Denver area (*The Lancet*, September 11, 1982), most of the victims had walked or crawled on freshly shampooed rugs. The basis of this observation is not yet known.

Life and Death
at the
Bellevue Stratford

Williamstown, Pennsylvania, a small Appalachian village (population 1,970 in the Bicentennial Year of 1976), hugs the side of Stoney Mountain, which forms the north rim of the Williams Valley some eighty miles northwest of Philadelphia. It is a community in economic distress. Along Market Street, low roofs extend from clapboard buildings out over the sidewalk; under them huddle many former business properties now bleak and empty. Economic problems are nothing new to the village. They have been a nearly perpetual feature of the community's life since the final closing of the nearby coal mines in the 1940s that left some 1,500 Williamstown people unemployed.

On Monday, August 2, 1976, however, Williamstown's distress was more than economic. Two previously healthy prominent male citizens, thirty-nine and forty-one years old, had died mysteriously within twenty-four hours, and Williamstown stirred with the kind of panic that used to accompany news of yet another mine disaster.

American Legion Post 239, whose three-story brick building is a prominent feature of the town's main street, has been commanded for more than twenty years by Richard Michael Dolan. Under "Dicko" Dolan's stewardship, Post finances have been carefully managed. The Post owns, among other things, the apartment buildings to either side of Legion Hall. It used $125,000 of its own money to build a large one-story factory building that it first leased to Clement Ball Shoe Corporation, then to AMP, Inc., an electronics firm that now employs some 350 people. It also donated to the state the six acres that is now home to the 131st Transportation Company of the Pennsylvania National Guard. Besides being a financial power in the community and a major benefactor of village charities, Post 239, with some 500 members, is also the social center with the only bar and the only dance floor in town, and a short-order counter where beer is 10 cents, hamburgers twice that.

Because of the central role Post 239 plays in Williamstown life, it was doubly shocking to the village when two of the younger Post members died so suddenly.

James T. Dolan, Dicko's cousin and the younger of the two victims, died on Sunday, August 1. Dicko Dolan had stood gravely by his cousin's final resting place in the Sacred Heart of Jesus Cemetery at the eastern end of Williamstown and lifted the American flag from the coffin before it was lowered into the ground. Jimmy's Legion cap sat forlornly atop a small American flag stuck in the freshly turned earth of his grave amid the floral wreaths.

John B. Ralph, Jr., known as J. B., had been owner and publisher of two local newspapers. He had also been a horn player, a baseball fan, and one of Williamstown's most popular citizens. A week before his death he had sponsored a dart-throwing contest at the Legion Hall—the darts champion of County Cork, Ireland, against all comers. J. B. had shaved his head, stuck cigarettes in both ears, and stood before the target while the Irish champion impaled each cigarette on a thrown dart. Prudently, J. B. had faced the dartboard rather than the unnerving sight of the sharp-tipped missiles hurtling toward him.

The following Thursday night J. B. was in the hospital, and by Monday he was dead. On Tuesday, August 3, after J. B.'s flag-draped bronze coffin made its final journey to Fairview Cemetery west of the village, Dicko Dolan presented the flag that had covered both coffins to J. B.'s mother.

Those who had driven with the funeral cortège up the tree-lined driveway of Fairview Cemetery were painfully aware that some of J. B.'s closest friends were absent for fear of contagion. When Dr. Stanley Doe's secretary went to a Little League baseball game later that week, she sat down next to some of her neighbors whose sons were also in the game. The other women hastily moved away, leaving the doctor's secretary hurt and alone. Dr. Doe had treated Jimmy Dolan.

For Dicko Dolan, a stocky, broad-shouldered man whose gray wavy hair is just beginning to thin, and whose face is usually punctuated with a cold cigar centered in his mouth like a lazy exclamation point, the sudden and mysterious death of his two friends, both Korean War veterans like himself, was a cruel shock. Why them, he asked himself? And why not me?

Throughout Pennsylvania, Legionnaires were dying. Ray Brennan had been the first. Ray, a former captain, was tall, slender, and graying at sixty-one. Since his retirement from the air force, he had lived quietly in the village of Towanda, some hundred miles from Philadelphia, where he was a deputy district commander of the Legion and bookkeeper for Post 42. On Tuesday, July 27, Ray Brennan had a fever, headache, pain in his chest, and difficulty breathing. His sister, Maise Travis, concerned because of her brother's history of heart disease, urged him to go to the hospital in Athens, a dozen miles away up the Susquehanna River toward the western New York State border. She finally prevailed, although, as she said, "We had to fight him all the way." His first night in the hospital, Ray Brennan died. The death certificate read, "Etiology unknown."

By the Saturday after Ray Brennan's death, six more Pennsylvania Legionnaires were dead. The day of Jimmy Dolan's death claimed another four, including the first woman, Mrs. Marie Tucker of Philadelphia. By Monday morning telephones were ringing ceaselessly in state and local public health offices throughout Pennsylvania, and in the administrative offices of the Centers for Disease Control (CDC) in Atlanta, whose cluster of tan and red brick buildings adjacent to Emory University is to the defense of the nation against disease what the drab, gray Pentagon is to the nation's military defense. The first call had come at 9:15 A.M., when Dr. Sidney Franklin of the Philadelphia Veterans Administration called Dr. Robert Craven at the CDC to report the deaths of four Legionnaires.

By late Monday, the death toll was still rising, sixty-three Legionnaires were hospitalized, and three epidemiologists from the CDC were flying through the late afternoon sun toward hot and windless Philadelphia to begin what would become the largest public health investigation in U.S. history, and one of the most frustrating.

Towanda didn't support much in the way of bright lights and night life, and Ray Brennan, like his fellow Legionnaires from other small towns in Pennsylvania, looked forward to the annual conventions of the Pennsylvania Department of the Legion that were held alternately in Pittsburgh and in Philadelphia. In 1976, the convention was in Philadelphia from July 21 to July 24. Ray Brennan, like all of the first eight Pennsylvania Legionnaires to die, had stayed in the headquarters hotel, the elegant seventy-two-year-old Bellevue Stratford, all marble and crystal and gilt trim, that Philadelphians proudly referred to as the "Grand Old Lady of Broad Street."

Guests of the Bellevue Stratford were housed in approximately 700 rooms. Each of the candidates for major offices in the Pennsylvania Legion had reserved a room, or a suite of rooms—the so-called hospitality suites, where drinks and snacks were served to the assembled Legionnaires. Besides these sources of free food and liquor, each district of the Pennsylvania Legion had its own hospitality suites, either in the Bellevue or elsewhere, as did many of the local posts. The convention activities included meetings for all delegates, a parade to Independence Hall, a testimonial dinner at the Benjamin Franklin Hotel seven blocks away, a dance in the Bellevue Stratford ballroom, committee meetings, regional caucuses, and a "Keystone Go-Getter" breakfast at the Bellevue Roof Garden.

The meeting rooms, nearby restaurants like the famous Bookbinders, hospitality suites, and topless bars were jammed by approximately 4,400 Legionnaires and a nearly equal number of Legion Auxiliary members, wives, and other family members and guests who descended on Philadelphia in late July. A steady stream of Legionnaires' cars drove to the Swinger's Sex Club across the Benjamin Franklin Bridge in New Jersey, which offered titillation not readily available in the staid City of Brotherly Love.

Soon the CDC had some 150 investigators working to track down the cause of what most of the press had dubbed "Legionnaires' disease," although *Time* magazine, even two years later, was still calling it the "Philly Killer." The CDC investigation was greatly supplemented by the skilled efforts of physicians and scientists in state, city, and private hospital and university laboratories throughout Pennsylvania. Time was of the essence. The following week the Forty-first Eucharistic Congress of Catholics was to meet in Philadelphia with headquarters at the Bellevue Stratford, and there were rumors that the Pope himself might attend. President Ford was to address the Congress there in that election year of 1976. The president requested hourly bulletins on the events in Pennsylvania.

There were two broad categories of agents that might have caused the illness suffered by so many Legionnaires who had in common only their visit to Philadelphia for the convention. The first was infectious agents: a bacterium, fungus, or virus. The second was toxic substances: poison, either deliberately administered or accidental contaminants in the food, water, or air.

Although the first eight victims of Legionnaires' disease to die had all stayed in the Bellevue Stratford, as the number of fatal cases increased so did the number of hotels involved. John Ralph, Jimmy Dolan, and Dicko Dolan had stayed at the Penn Center Holiday Inn seven blocks from the Bellevue, while other victims had stayed at the Ben Franklin, headquarters for the Legion Auxiliary, or elsewhere in the dozen or so hotels in the downtown area. But all the victims seemed to have in common the fact that they had either spent time in the lobby of the Bellevue Stratford, in its meeting rooms, or on the sidewalk outside while, for example, watching the parade to Independence Hall. So, although the other hotels weren't overlooked, the search for the agent of Legionnaires' disease centered on the "Grand Old Lady of Broad Street."

The nature of the illness made a toxic agent seem unlikely. The high fever experienced by the victims of Legionnaires' disease (up to 108° F in some cases) was characteristic of an infectious disease. The investigators knew of no toxic agent that caused a fever in humans or laboratory animals that would not have been instantly apparent to the victims by its strange taste or disagreeable odor. So the search was initially directed toward the most likely culprit—a fungal, viral, or bacterial agent.

Most bacteria and fungi are free-living agents capable of growth in suitable liquid or solid media. Samples of tissues and fluids from victims of the disease were examined under the microscope for traces of unusual organisms and then divided among containers of more than a dozen different solid and liquid media designed to distinguish fungi from bacteria, and subclasses of bacteria and fungi from one another by their characteristic growth patterns, as well as to provide additional material with which to carry out further diagnostic chemical reactions.

Viruses, unlike most bacteria and fungi, are completely parasitic organisms unable to grow except inside the cells of a suitable host. Many viruses, such as the influenza strains discussed earlier, grow well in the cells that surround a chicken embryo after a certain point in gestation and are shed into the egg fluid. Other viruses grow best in cultures of mammalian cells taken from, for example, monkey kidney or human embryos, or in newborn mice or guinea pigs.

The investigators also had to consider agents like the small bacteria called rickettsiae that, like viruses, grow only as intracellular parasites and can consequently be isolated from infected eggs, mammalian cell cultures, or the tissues of infected guinea pigs. Rickettsiae can be readily distinguished from viruses by the fact that they are visible in an ordinary microscope while viruses require the many thousand-fold greater magnification (and higher resolving power) of the electron microscope to be detectable.

The search was complicated by the fact that bacteria and fungi are always found in or on the normal human body, whereas viruses, although never normally present in human body fluids, may easily arise from contamination of the sample by virus-laden air or water or by viruses already present in the inoculated cells or culture media.

A few days after the research effort had begun in half a dozen laboratories, the results began to come in and were communicated through a command post set up in a large ground-floor room of the Philadelphia Health Department Office in the Municipal Service Building just four blocks from the Bellevue Stratford. Known bacteria were quickly eliminated by the collaborative effort in the local, state, private, and CDC laboratories. There was no evidence for a new variety of bacteria as a cause of Legionnaires' disease.

It took another day or so to eliminate the slower-growing yeasts and molds (fungi) as possible infectious agents. Most of the scientists involved in the search were betting that a virus was the causative agent. In addition to the attempts to culture such an agent from egg amniotic fluid and cell cultures, samples of tissue and body fluids of the dead Legionnaires were examined for viruses in electron microscopes in several research centers. The investigators soon found that there seemed to be no unusual viral particles in any of the samples, although that did not rule out a virus that was indistinguishable by appearance alone from a common viral agent. Naturally, the possibility of swine flu was very much on everyone's mind. It had been only five months since the death from swine flu of the young recruit at Fort Dix, and the country was in the throes of trying to organize a program of mass immunization against that disease by early fall (see chapters 2 and 3).

By Wednesday evening, August 4, a light rain was falling in Philadelphia, a legacy of Hurricane Belle that had swept up the coast the day before, and the spirits of the investigators in Pennsylvania and elsewhere were falling as well. By then, twenty persons had died of Legionnaires' disease, including two women (another woman would die the next day). One hundred thirty other victims were hospitalized, and still no one had a firm clue as to what the agent of Legionnaires' disease might be. It was neither a known bacterium nor a fungus. It was certainly not swine flu virus; it was not an influenza virus of any sort and, in fact, it did not appear to be a virus at all, although the earliest four autopsies on victims of the disease had indicated that severe viral pneumonia was the cause of death. If it was none of those agents, then what was it? Weary scientists in Philadelphia, Pittsburgh, Atlanta, and elsewhere turned that question over and over in their minds, examining it from every angle, and, finding nothing they had not already considered and eliminated, went to bed hoping that morning would bring fresh inspiration.

On August 5, Pennsylvania's governor, Milton J. Shapp, announced publicly that flu was not the cause of the epidemic and that toxicological studies by the CDC were beginning.[1] Jay Satz, M.D., a virologist at the Pennsylvania State Health

Department laboratory in Philadelphia, was quoted as saying, "If this is a virus, it is a very unusual virus." He went on: "I am treating this organism in my laboratory as an extremely dangerous one . . . I have to consider my own life and the lives of my technical people."[2]

That same evening, on CBS Evening News, Legionnaires around Pennsylvania told stories that echoed the experience of Dr. Doe's secretary in Williamstown when she was shunned at the Little League game because her employer had treated Jimmy Dolan. Martin Baker from Harrisburg was not ill but, as he told TV interviewer Gary Shepard, his neighbors and some Legionnaires were avoiding him because he had been at the Philadelphia convention. Ray Weaver reported that members of his Legion Post moved when he sat down next to them, and one said, "Don't come near me. Stay away!"[3]

The next night, Charles Murphy of ABC Evening News interviewed Dr. Sencer, the director of the Center for Disease Control, who verified that the agent of the Philadelphia epidemic was not flu of any kind, neither was it a fungus or a bacterium. There was no evidence for a viral agent, and, as Dr. Sencer admitted, the next phase of the investigation—the search for a toxic agent—would be even tougher. On NBC that evening, another CDC spokesman stated that the agent had to be a toxin and that the Center was getting 3,000 calls every hour on Legionnaires' disease.

Many professional students of epidemics wear a small silver lapel pin in the shape of a shoe sole with a hole in it. It is a tribute to the time-honored discipline of "shoe-leather" epidemiology, the tedious accumulation of facts about an epidemic until a pattern finally begins to emerge. In the United States most epidemiologists are, or were, part of the Epidemic Intelligence Service (EIS) of the CDC. Before long, twenty EIS officers, mostly young physicians, fanned out across Pennsylvania. Donning sterile gloves, gowns, and masks, they interviewed sick Legionnaires in their hospital beds, asking them what convention events they had attended, where they had stayed in Philadelphia, what and where they had eaten and drunk, whom they had roomed with, eaten with, or talked to. Later, a two-page questionnaire was sent to members of the 1,002 Posts of the Pennsylvania Legion to elicit the same information from all those who had been in Philadelphia.

The EIS officers next examined hospital charts, talked to the attending physicians, the victims' friends and families, and anyone else who might offer a helpful fact about the victims' habits and their activities during the convention. In addition to the interviews, every one of the state's more than 300 hospitals was checked by telephone for information on cases of Legionnaires' disease. It was an imposing effort. But it didn't stop the dying.

Fortunately, the epidemic was slacking off. After the middle of the first week in August, new hospitalizations for Legionnaires' disease and reports of fatal cases began to decline, although it was the end of the month before public health officials were reasonably certain that the onslaught had passed.

To begin to understand the epidemic that had struck central Philadelphia during July and August 1976, epidemiologists first had to decide what constituted a case of the disease. They settled on a definition that required that a victim of Legionnaires' disease had to have fallen sick between July 1 and August 18 with an illness that included a cough, a fever of 102° F or higher, or a lower fever if accompanied by X-ray evidence of pneumonia. (The filling of portions of the lung with fluid, characteristic of pneumonia, causes those portions to appear darker in X-ray photographs than if they were filled, as they normally are, with air.) There was also an epidemiological criterion, namely, that the victim had either attended the Legion convention or had entered the Bellevue Stratford between July 1 and the onset of his or her illness.

Several victims contracted a disease that appeared to be clinically identical to Legionnaires' disease, although they had neither attended the Legion convention nor been in the

Bellevue Stratford. These people were grouped separately under the provisional category of Broad Street pneumonia if they had been within one block of the Bellevue between July 1 and the start of their illness. With the definitions of Legionnaires' disease and Broad Street pneumonia agreed upon, the collection of cases could be examined in more detail by the epidemiologists for clues as to their sources.

There were 182 cases that met the definition of Legionnaires' disease; 40 of the victims were women. Patients ranged in age from three to eighty-two years; the mean age was nearly fifty-five. Jimmy Dolan, at thirty-nine, was the youngest person to die. Only 4 percent of the Legionnaires and their family members and guests attending the convention became ill; 16 percent of the cases (about one in six) were fatal; those who died were ill for about a week before their deaths. A candlemaker's convention just before the Legion convention supplied two victims of Legionnaires' disease; a magician's convention just before the candlemakers supplied another; and the Eucharist Congress that followed the Legionnaires into the Bellevue Stratford produced nine more. The first two victims from the Congress were a fifty-four-year-old priest, Monsignor John F. Donnelly, and a thirty-eight-year-old musician, both of whom had stayed at the Bellevue. The unfortunate musician's name was Louis Fortunate.

Gradually, a composite picture of the typical victim of Legionnaires' disease emerged. Although only 4 out of every 100 persons attending the Legion convention contracted the disease, it struck a far greater proportion of the older veterans, particularly if they had stayed at the Bellevue Stratford.

Of the twenty-nine fatal cases that met the criteria for Legionnaires' disease, sixteen of the victims had stayed at the Bellevue, and six others had stayed at the Penn Central Holiday Inn. Jane Palmer, sixty-four, a member of the Legion Auxiliary, had only stood on the sidewalk in front of the Bellevue to watch the Friday morning parade.

The victims of Legionnaires' disease had spent more time

in the lobby of the Bellevue Stratford (nearly twice as much) and on the sidewalk in front of the hotel than had those who escaped the illness. Some, like Jane Palmer, had done no more than stand in front of the hotel to watch the parade on the humid, smoggy Friday before the convention ended. There was no evidence of person-to-person spread. Legionnaires' disease, whatever it was, was at least not contagious.

Cigarette smokers were more than three times as likely to have acquired Legionnaires' disease as were those who smoked pipes or cigars, or who didn't smoke at all.

There was no correlation, however, between contracting Legionnaires' disease and whether a Legionnaire had drunk alcoholic beverages, eaten in any of the many restaurants and bars around the Bellevue Stratford, put ice in a drink, or gone to the various hospitality suites (although the ill delegates visited half again as many hospitality suites as those who did not become ill) and a greater proportion of victims had visited a fourteenth-floor hospitality suite than among those who remained well. There was also no correlation between where in the Bellevue Stratford their rooms were located or with whom they had shared them. Among the ill delegates to the Legion convention, a greater proportion had drunk the water at the Bellevue Stratford than of those delegates who remained well.

Broad Street pneumonia claimed thirty-nine victims; five cases were fatal. Two thirds of the cases were in males; the average age of victims of Broad Street pneumonia was slightly more than fifty years.

When the epidemiologists tabulated the dates on which the victims became ill, it was clear that what had occurred was a common source epidemic—that is, the victims had been exposed for a relatively short period to a common source of their illness, after which the source had temporarily ceased to exist. One victim of Legionnaires' disease became ill on July 20, another on the 22nd. On successive days there were five, eleven, twenty-five, twenty-four, twenty-five, and twenty-two new cases. Then the numbers declined sharply. None of the victims became ill on August 4, 5, 7, or 8, after which there was another spurt of activity with thirteen new cases, the last of which began on August 16.

Of the 169 cases of Legionnaires' disease in the major outbreak, 16 occurred in those not attending the Legion convention. None of the fourteen victims of the disease who became ill after August 6 had been at the Legion meeting. Broad Street pneumonia followed a similar pattern, with a major and a later minor peak, and none of the victims of Broad Street pneumonia had taken part in the Legion meeting.

Considering the age distribution of those attending the Legion convention and the current mortality statistics for Pennsylvania, the epidemiological teams laboriously calculated that the death rate between July 27 and August 16 was more than seven times that expected—additional evidence that an epidemic had occurred. Exposure to the source of infection, whatever it may have been, had occurred, at the very least, on July 22 and 23, and again some time during the intervals August 1–3 and August 6–9. Although the season of the epidemic and some of its characteristics suggested an insect-borne disease, the victims of Legionnaires' disease had not noticed insect bites.

While the lights burned late over the desks of the epidemiologists as they gradually inked in the portrait of the epidemic, laboratory studies of potential poisons and infectious agents were also going forward. By August 16, seventeen potentially toxic metals had been eliminated, including mercury, arsenic, and cadmium. Tissue samples from the dead Legionnaires were ultimately analyzed for more than thirty metallic elements and for a large number of toxic organic compounds. The serum from victims was tested for antibodies against seventy-seven infectious agents; thirteen different animal host systems for viruses were tested in an effort to isolate a viral agent. More than a dozen kinds of media that would allow the growth of bacteria or fungi were tested, and samples were examined with a variety of stains and by both light and electron microscopy for the presence of an infectious agent.

Rickettsiae, among which are the agents of Q fever and Rocky Mountain spotted fever, were sought for, but in vain. Serum from victims of Legionnaires' disease was also tested, frequently by more than one method, for antibodies to more than a dozen viruses, eleven rickettsiae, pathogenic fungi, spirochetes, parasitic worms, amoebae, and the group of small bacteria called chlamydia that, like the rickettsiae, grow only inside animal cells and that cause diseases like psittacosis (parrot fever).

After countless hours of work by some of the most sophisticated scientists in federal, state, city, university, and private research organizations, the CDC called together a group of a dozen well-known pathologists from around the country to review the slides of the tissues of human and animal victims of the disease, and the results of the many analyses made for both toxins and infectious agents. In late August, the panel, after examining the vast amount of data collected, concluded that the agent could be a toxic chemical or a virus, but that it was certainly not a bacterium.

Was it poison? Some Legionnaires thought so. The Vietnam War was not long past, and feeling against anything military still ran high in some quarters. Hippies had picketed the Bellevue Stratford headquarters of the Legion convention, and the presence of the grimy, ragged, long-haired youths had infuriated many Legionnaires. It was freely suggested that hippies had somehow poisoned the water at the Bellevue Stratford.

On August 8, an FBI spokesman denied the report made on a San Francisco radio station that the FBI and the CIA were investigating the theft of a toxic substance from the army's chemical and biological warfare laboratory at Fort Detrick, Maryland.

Then there was the mysterious "glassy-eyed" man. George Chiavetta, a Legionnaire from Lawson, Pennsylvania, later testified before the House Subcommittee on Consumer Protection and Finance that he had seen a glassy-eyed stranger in a royal blue suit on three different occasions during the convention. He had overheard the man saying: "It's too late. You won't be saved. The Legionnaires are doomed." Chiavetta said that four other members of his Legion Post also saw the stranger at convention functions and an Identikit photo of the mystery man appeared in the *National Enquirer* and in Associated Press dispatches to newspapers all over the country. According to Chiavetta, who was described by those who knew him as sober and reliable, the glassy-eyed man also had a bag of some sort hanging from the inside of his suit coat. A tube from this bag ran across his chest and, apparently, down his left sleeve to a rolled-up newspaper, which he pointed at the Legionnaires. The "glassy-eyed" man was never found.

Health officials had plenty of suggestions from the public about the cause of Legionnaires' disease. Dr. Harvey Friedman, director of the diagnostic virology laboratory at Philadelphia's Children's Hospital, got a call telling him that the cause of Legionnaires' disease was contaminated soda. "I know," said the caller, "I drank a bottle with viral pneumonia in it. I got the bottle!"[4] Dicko Dolan and his buddies had complained about dank vapors seeping from the air-conditioning vents in their eighth-floor room at the Penn Center Holiday Inn and unusual wet spots on the carpet. Newspaper offices across the country got calls from people who felt that Legionnaires' disease was a retaliation by the Martians for the landing of the Viking I spacecraft on their planet late in July.

A black minister wrote the Philadelphia Department of Health to suggest that the disease came from outer space and that it would return but that next time it would primarily affect children. A Pennsylvania dentist, in a nearly incoherent letter signed Former Air Force Person, blamed the whole thing on the Jews; another writer pointed out that it could only be cholera caused by the Legionnaires eating pork from pigs with hog cholera that, with the connivance of corrupt state and federal health officials, had not been destroyed but instead sent to market. Unfortunately for this theory, human cholera is caused by a bacterium and affects only humans, while hog cholera is caused by a virus and affects only pigs.

The U.S. Labor Party put out a two-page "Fact Sheet" on the Philadelphia "Killer Fever" that was anything but factual. The Labor Party had decided that the disease was swine flu, but that this fact was being suppressed because of political pressure from Sen. Edward Kennedy, along with his colleagues Senators Schweiker, Javits, and Mondale, who had opposed the swine flu program. The outbreak of "swine flu" in Philadelphia would expose the senators' position "for the genocidal policy it in fact is," according to the Labor Party. This "political pressure" on CDC had caused the director of the CDC to make statements "both medically incompetent and dishonest," that "fly in the face of accepted medical opinion. These statements are accordingly criminally irresponsible," and so on.

The prize for the most imaginative theory of Legionnaires' disease should perhaps go to someone who signed himself James Jackson, General, U.S. Army Counter-Intelligence Corps, ASN 09360672, from Sherman Oaks, California. Jackson's theory, as explained in his letter to the Philadelphia Health Department, was that "the 38 Penn. Legionnaires" had been murdered by Frank Sinatra, who had also murdered John F. Kennedy, Howard Hughes, Rosalind Russell, and President Ford's brother, and had forced Ford to give the Panama Canal and Rhodesia to the Communists. Less amusing is the letter's last sentence, which reports that "Van Nuys (California) Am. Legion Post #193 has formed a vigalante [sic] committee and intends to fire bomb, with rockets, the White House, the Van Nuys News, Courthouse and First Baptist Church; and KGIL Radio of San Fernando, CA."

All these theories were interesting, amusing, and sometimes frightening. But the investigators were searching for something that they could weigh, measure, or photograph.

From the earliest moments of the investigation, samples of food, water, ice, carpets, draperies, wallpaper, glasses, and other appurtenances of the Bellevue Stratford and other hotels and restaurants where the Legionnaires had gathered had been taken for sophisticated chemical analysis on the chance that the agent of the disease might be a toxic chemical, whether deliberately planted or not.

Another investigation of the drinking water (and the water used in the air-conditioning system) at the Bellevue Stratford revealed that the water was typical of that in large urban areas, that is, it contained more than two dozen toxic organic compounds, some of them known carcinogens, albeit in very small amounts. Neither the range of compounds discovered nor their concentrations was particularly unusual—in itself a horrifying conclusion, but one of no particular relevance to Legionnaires' disease. Meanwhile, the death toll had mounted to 29, 2 of them women, and 151 others had been hospitalized with the malady.

In Pittsburgh, the Alleghany County coroner, Dr. Cyril H. Wecht, made another of the allegations for which he had become justly famous. He had found crystals of oxalate in the kidneys of two of the three victims of Legionnaires' disease he had examined. He suggested that this might have resulted from the ingestion of ethylene glycol, or diethylene glycol, common ingredients in antifreeze, hand lotion, and many other preparations. Dr. Wecht's suggestion was that it could have come from moonshine drunk by the Legionnaires.[5] A number of other explanations were equally probable, among them the chance that the victims took large quantities of vitamin C, which leads to the formation of oxalic acid kidney stones in some people.

While all this was going on, a thirtieth victim of the disease was about to succumb. Since the widely publicized epidemic in late July, occupancy at the Bellevue Stratford had dropped to a catastrophic 8 percent or less. The Houston Astros and the San Francisco Giants had canceled reservations, six conventions switched to Miami Beach, and another six were negotiating for a similar move. Although the House of Delegates of the Pennsylvania Medical Society continued its plan to meet at the Bellevue for three days in mid-September, the AMA was considering switching the meeting it had scheduled for December. Governor and Mrs. Shapp stayed overnight at the Bellevue Stratford as a gesture of support, but the hotel was still losing $10,000 every day.

In mid-November 1976 a meeting of public health investigators took place in the pink- and gold-domed Cameo Room atop the Bellevue Stratford to review what was known about the origin of Legionnaires' disease. Speaker after speaker presented convincing evidence that the agent was not a bacterium, not a virus, not a fungus, not a toxic chemical. America's disease detectives, among the finest in the world, were baffled and humiliated by the disease, and the meeting ended with solemn statements that the cause might never be known. Then, on Thursday, November 18, three days after the meeting of public health officials, the "Grand Old Lady of Broad Street" closed its doors. A few days later a sign appeared: "For Sale. Bellevue Stratford, Philadelphia's Finest Hotel. Call 854-1550. Albert M. Greenfield & Co., Inc." A call to Albert M. Greenfield & Co., Inc., revealed that the asking price for "Philadelphia's Finest Hotel" was a mere $10.5 million. The hotel had cost $10 million to build in 1904!

On December 3, 1976, the respected magazine *Science*, published by the American Association for the Advancement of Science, ran an article in its News and Comments section entitled: "Legion Fever: Postmortem on an Investigation That Failed." The article, written by Barbara J. Culliton, referred to the increasingly widespread view that no one would ever know what caused Legion fever. It was a spectacular admission of the failure of American science in one of its rare appearances in the full glare of the floodlights at center stage. The *Science* article pointed out that Representative John M. Murphy (D.-N.Y.)—whose committee on

Consumer Protection and Finance had written the recently enacted Toxic Substances Control Act—had declared in a "confidential" report of October 28: "It is totally unacceptable that in a country of 220 million people, supposedly with the most advanced technology in the world, we find ourselves in the position of not knowing what happened in Philadelphia and, even worse, not being in a position to prevent it from happening again." Congressman Murphy referred to the entire investigation as a "fiasco"—a popular word applied to public health matters in the fall of 1976—and criticized the CDC for "poor communications, an initial misdirection of resources almost bordering on tunnel vision toward swine flu, and a decided lack of organization."

The report also quoted Dr. F. William Sunderman, Jr., of the University of Connecticut School of Medicine, as saying that the cause of the epidemic was a saboteur who had somehow exposed the Legionnaires to nickel carbonyl, a colorless, odorless, and highly poisonous gas. Congressman Murphy concluded: "It appears to be the consensus of opinion that the failure to save, take and keep free of contamination the tissues of victims of this epidemic is clearly the reason that ultimate resolution of the cause of Legionnaires' disease may never be found."

It was uncertain whose opinions, in addition to John Murphy's, were part of this consensus. Dr. Sunderman, part of a father-son team of experts in nickel chemistry and toxicology, promptly replied that the report misconstrued and misquoted his views. And it was by no means clear that the way victims' tissues had been handled prevented the cause of the disease from ever being found. What was clear was that many toxicologists were unhappy about the way the investigation had been conducted.

In early August 1976, the CDC investigators were not thinking "toxicology," they were thinking "infectious agent," and so were most of their collaborators. The administration of the CDC was vulnerable to the charge of neglecting toxicology, and they knew it. Dr. Sencer was unavailable for comment to Barbara Culliton, *Science's* reporter—another of the CDC's public relations failures of 1976—and a number of toxicologists who tried to offer advice to the CDC in connection with Legionnaires' disease had been unable to get through to the agency and were annoyed about it. But, as Renate Kimbrough, M.D., a CDC toxicologist, later explained: "I was getting a hundred calls a day. I was trying to make studies that I hoped would help solve the problem. I could either work or I could return telephone calls. I chose to work."[6]

On the other hand, once the investigators settled in and it became increasingly doubtful that an infectious agent was involved, toxicological investigations were carried out under the auspices of the CDC, but to no avail. As Dr. H. Bruce Dull, one of the epidemiologists at the CDC, later put it: "It is just so hard to accept the fact that in 1976 there are some things we don't know."[7] That was true of both the scientists and the politicians, but it did not deflect the storm of criticism that rained down on CDC's Atlanta headquarters from those who demanded either an instantaneous solution to the Legionnaires' disease mystery—*à la* Marcus Welby, M.D.—or, failing that, a suitable scapegoat.

At the CDC, where the staff still smarted under the double lash of the cancelation of the swine flu immunization program and the failure to isolate the agent of Legionnaires' disease, Christmas 1976 was far less festive than in other years since, after the expenditure of 90,000 man hours and $2 million, the cause of Legionnaires' disease remained unknown. Reminders of the unsuccessful investigation were everywhere. Even at cocktail parties CDC staffers were asked if they had solved the mystery of Legionnaires' disease yet, and if not, why not?

Dr. David Fraser, the young Harvard-trained physician who had very recently been put in charge of the epidemiological part of the investigation, had collected progress reports from his team, written up a summary—called EPI-2 since it was the second such summary of the status of the Legionnaires' disease study—and personally distributed it to a large number of his CDC colleagues, including Charles Shepard, M.D., who ran the leprosy and rickettsia laboratory of the Center.

The laboratory of Dr. Shepard and his colleagues is in Building Seven on the CDC campus. No one could then enter Building Seven unless he or she had had a smallpox vaccination within the past year. Legionnaires' disease seemed a far cry from the leprosy and Rocky Mountain spotted fever (tick-borne typhus) that were the subject of most of the work of Dr. Shepard and his colleagues. But Dr. Fraser, with his casual dress and boyish good looks, was also thorough and conscientious; he wanted everyone to know where the investigation stood.

The Monday after Christmas, December 27, was a quiet day at the CDC. Many of the staff were gone, using up the vacation they would otherwise lose at the end of the calendar year. But one of Dr. Shepard's colleagues, Dr. Joseph McDade, a square-jawed, mustachioed microbiologist, was in the lab with nothing particular to do that day. Joe McDade, thirty-seven, had been at the CDC for only fifteen months after spending four years working on epidemic typhus in Egypt and Ethiopia. He sat down to look over the copy of EPI-2 that David Fraser had dropped off. McDade had looked for rickettsiae in the specimens from victims of Legionnaires' disease in August but had found nothing. Other workers in the infectious disease branch housed in Building Seven had looked for bacteria, fungi, and viruses, with equal lack of success.

Two statements in EPI-2 about Legionnaires' disease triggered a chain of thought in Dr. McDade's mind. The first statement was that victims of the disease aften had elevated levels of a liver enzyme called serum glutamic-oxalacetic transaminase (abbreviated SGOT) in their blood. This was not surprising; many of the victims were heavy drinkers, and heavy drinking, like many other things, causes breakdown of liver cells and release of liver enzymes into the blood. But elevated levels of SGOT are also characteristic of rickettsial diseases. It was also reported in EPI-2 that Q fever, an insect-borne rickettsial disease, could not be absolutely ruled out as a cause of Legion fever. It then occurred to Dr. McDade that perhaps the agent of the disease was a new form of rickettsia, although none had been identified since before he had been born. In any case, he reached for the box on his desk that contained slides from the earlier investigation of the Philadelphia outbreak and took another look.

All the slides had been examined earlier for an average of about five minutes apiece. This is ordinarily enough time for an experienced person to detect whether the sample on the slide contains organisms. Dr. McDade spent thirty minutes looking at the first slide, millimeter by millimeter. This time Joe McDade was not looking for the usual rickettsiae. He was looking for anything out of the ordinary. And he found it.

In a single field, he suddenly saw a cluster of red rods inside the spleen cells from a guinea pig that had been infected with lung tissues from a dead Legionnaire. He had never seen anything like it before, and he carefully noted the coordinates of the cluster from the calibrated microscope stage so he could find the same place again. Then he looked at the rest of the slide, and at many more besides.

The next day, McDade returned to the slide on which he had seen the clump of organisms and soon realized just how difficult they were to find. Even with the coordinates of the clump of organisms written in his notebook, he had to search for a long time before finding the red rods.

In August, others of Dr. Shepard's group had tried to grow up rickettsiae from Legionnaires' tissue samples by injecting them into eggs after treating the samples with penicillin and streptomycin to keep down the growth of common bacteria with which the samples might be contaminated. No rickettsiae grew in the inoculated eggs. Now Dr. McDade decided to inject tissue into eggs without first adding antimicrobials, so that the mysterious red rods, whatever they were, would have a better chance to grow. As an extra precaution he ordered eggs from chickens that had never received antimicrobial drugs.

On Wednesday, January 5, the embryos in the eggs that he had injected on New Year's Eve with spleen samples from guinea pigs ill with Legionnaires' disease began to die. Most bacteria would have killed the embryos in forty-eight hours or less, so the fact that the embryos had lived so long was consistent with the idea that the organisms were an unusual rickettsia. Joe McDade removed the amniotic fluid from the eggs, carried out the Giménez staining procedure that had yielded the organisms stained with red aniline dyes, and sat down at his microscope. The egg fluid swarmed with blunt red rods.

Were they the agent of Legionnaires' disease? If they were, then sera from Legionnaires recovering from the disease should have antibodies to these organisms. Dr. McDade needed such serum samples urgently.

Saving serum and tissue samples is a CDC tradition. In several dozen freezers are over a quarter million vials of serum from disease outbreaks going back more than thirty years. By now, Dr. Charles Shepard and a few of Dr. McDade's other colleagues knew what he had found. Dr. Shepard used his considerable influence to obtain convalescent serum from five victims of Legionnaires' disease, as well as serum taken from the same people early in their illness. Martha Redus, an expert in what is called the indirect fluorescent antibody test, exposed molecules of a fluorescent antibody to the proteins in the test sera. To samples of Joseph McDade's organisms on a microscope slide were added a few drops of the convalescent serum, then the fluorescent antibody. If the disease that the Legionnaires had suffered was caused by Dr.

McDade's rods, then the antibodies that appeared in their blood while they were recovering from the disease should bind tightly to the rods, and to the fluorescent antibody, while other fluorescent proteins in the serum would be washed away.

After allowing time for the fluorescent antibodies to attach to the organisms, Redus washed the slide free of contaminating fluorescent protein and dried it. Meanwhile Joe McDade stood by, exhausted. He had been sleeping poorly for a week and was, by turns, too tired and too excited to be of any use in the laboratory. The slides wouldn't be ready to examine until early evening, so McDade went home while Martha Redus continued her painstaking work.

Joe McDade was equally ineffectual at home. He had no appetite and couldn't concentrate on anything. At 8:00 p.m. that Friday evening, January 7, the telephone rang. It was Martha Redus. Two of the five serum samples from convalescent victims of Legionnaires' disease contained fluorescent antibodies that bound tightly to the blunt red rods McDade had first seen the Monday after Christmas, while the serum taken at the beginning of the victims' illness did not. This positive result in two samples was far more significant than the negative result in the other three because some people, especially those in poor health, do not form antibodies vigorously. In addition, as was discovered later, antibody formation may not occur until six weeks after the beginning of Legionnaires' disease, and many of the samples of convalescent serum had been taken from one to four weeks after the victim became ill.

What about Broad Street pneumonia? In the next few days the indirect fluorescent antibody test showed that two of four samples of serum from patients convalescing from Broad Street pneumonia reacted with McDade's rods. Before long it was certain—Broad Street pneumonia and Legionnaires' disease were the same thing. This meant that there had been, in all, 221 cases of Legionnaires' disease in Philadelphia, of which 34 were fatal, and the term "Broad Street pneumonia" passed into oblivion.

On Tuesday afternoon, January 18, the discovery of the agent of Legionnaires' disease—later christened *Legionella pneumophila*—was announced at a CDC press conference. Neither Dr. McDade nor Dr. Shepard was happy about the announcement. They felt that further tests should be done to rule out even the slightest chance that the discovery was a fluke. But leaks to the press were a virtual certainty once word had gone through the CDC that the agent had been discovered, and Dr. Sencer made the announcement that day to an auditorium overflowing with people from the news media and some 300 cheering CDC employees. By then it was almost certain that the organism was not a rickettsiae but rather a new type of gram-negative bacterium.

Because it was now possible to recognize the bacterium, the next steps were to grow it in artificial media and to determine which antimicrobial drugs were most effective against it.

There were many other questions as well. Was *Legionella pneumophila* a newly evolved organism, and how had it come to attack the Legionnaires and others in Philadelphia? The first question was easily answered; the answer to the second is still not completely clear.

To some of the downy-cheeked young accountants in the Office of Management and Budget, the CDC's thirty-seven freezers filled with ancient serum samples must have seemed the height of scientific foolishness and waste. But, as many times before, the massive collection quickly proved its worth.

On Sunday, July 18, 1965, a drenching rainstorm had struck Washington, D.C., accompanied by winds of nearly fifty miles an hour. On the more than seventy-five-year-old campus of St. Elizabeth's Hospital—a huge general psychiatric institution across the Potomac from Washington National

Airport—several trees were uprooted, and dust from excavations for a new sprinkling system was blown in the windows of the hospital buildings, which were not air-conditioned. By Tuesday, July 27, an epidemic of undiagnosed respiratory illness began among the patients of St. Elizabeth's. Ultimately, there were at least 81 cases and 14 deaths among the hospital's approximately 6,000 patients. Of the eighty-one known victims of the disease, seventy-four either had ground privileges (that is, they were free to move about portions of the 350-acre campus of the hospital) and/or they slept by open windows. In either case, these privileges were transformed into a curse because those patients suffered greater exposure to the dust blowing from the excavations. The attack rates of the disease were ten times higher in buildings close to the excavations than in those far away. Although the outbreak was carefully investigated by CDC officers at the time, the disease agent was never identified.

Dr. Charles Shepard was struck immediately by the similarity between the St. Elizabeth's outbreak and Legionnaires' disease. Serum samples taken from the patients at the Washington hospital were in the CDC freezers. The twenty-six samples available were quickly tested for the presence of antibody to *Legionella pneumophila (L. pneumophila)*. Twenty-two of the twenty-six samples of serum from patients convalescing from the mysterious illness glowed with the yellow-green fluorescence of fluorescein when examined under ultraviolet light; most of the sera taken early in the disease did not. Legionnaires' disease had struck St. Elizabeth's Hospital eleven years before the Legion convention in Philadelphia.

There was another mysterious illness in the 1960s that had been a thorn in the flesh of CDC investigators. During the first three weeks of June 1968, the ground alongside the one-story County Health Department building in Pontiac, Michigan, was regraded and paved. This operation raised clouds of dust that periodically enveloped the brown brick building. An air conditioner, defective in both design and operation, also contributed to the explosion of an unknown disease in the Health Department building.

On Tuesday evening, July 9, 1968, three Epidemic Intelligence Service officers from the CDC who had been sent to investigate the unidentified disease had come down with it as well. Three more young physicians sent from the CDC to replace them had also contracted the disease. Although "Pontiac fever," as it was dubbed, resembled Legionnaires' disease in some ways, there were important differences. It was not primarily respiratory; it was self-limiting, that is, it went away by itself without treatment; it lasted only two to five days; none of the 144 victims died; and only one was hospitalized. Forty-nine of those stricken had only visited the Health Department building and some of those had been inside less than half an hour. Pontiac fever was also unique in attacking 95 percent of the staff of the Health Department building, compared with the 4 percent attack rate of Legionnaires' disease in Philadelphia. The serum samples from the Pontiac outbreak had again been stored in the CDC freezers. They were tested for antibodies to *L. pneumophila*, and—marvelous to relate—Pontiac fever, though very different in many important ways from Legionnaires' disease, was shown to be caused by the same, or a very similar, organism.

The observations on Pontiac fever led to another discovery. On Monday, July 30, 1973, ten previously healthy young men spent nine hours cleaning, with compressed air lines and hoses, a huge steam turbine condenser (21 feet long and 12 feet in diameter) alongside the James River in Virginia. In the next three or four days, all ten had become ill with symptoms like those of Pontiac fever. And, sure enough, when the serum from those men was taken from the CDC serum bank and tested, samples from eight of the ten men were found to contain antibodies to the Legionnaires' disease bacterium.

The CDC's serum collection was international and so, it soon devoloped, was Legionnaires' disease. Out of a tour group of 252 Scots returning to Glasgow from Spain in late July 1973, 164 were ill. All the sick tourists had stayed in the same hotel in Benidorm on the Mediterranean coast of Spain. One of the tourists, a fifty-four-year-old man, died on the flight home. Two more men, aged fifty and sixty-two, re-spectively, died in Glasgow. Two other Scottish tourists, a sixty-four-year-old man and a fifty-one-year-old woman, re-turning from Spain four years later (one from the same hotel used by the earlier group) also died shortly after their return to Glasgow. All these cases were identified retroactively as Legionnaires' disease; six members of the hotel staff in Beni-dorm had high serum levels of antibody to *L. pneumophila*. In May 1976, a twenty-one-year-old Glasgow woman died of the same disease, acquired in Scotland and diagnosed retro-actively by Dr. William Cherry of the CDC.

A fatal case of Legionnaires' disease occurred in Notting-ham, England, in June 1976, when a forty-two-year-old woman died. By April 1978, there had been fifteen cases reported in Nottingham (the youngest victim was twenty-four), with nearly all the cases occurring in people living in the same small area of the community. Nineteen other cases had been reported from elsewhere in England and Wales.

At Oxford University Medical Centre, the Legion bacillus was isolated from water in the shower of a kidney transplant unit in the summer of 1979 after two women, aged twenty-nine and fifty-four, respectively, had acquired Legionnaires' disease while in the unit. Chlorination of the water, known to inhibit bacteral growth, had only a temporary effect; the organism was isolated from the showers again nine months later.

Cases of Legionnaires' disease have also appeared in Sweden (sixty-seven in a single city in one month), as well as in Italy, Yugoslavia, Canada, Denmark, Greece, Israel, Norway, The Netherlands, the German Federal Republic,

France, Portugal, South Africa, and Australia. The agent of Legionnaires' disease exists in soil and water throughout the world and probably always has. At present it is known to have caused eighteen epidemics, five of which preceded the Bicentennial convention of Pennsylvania Legionnaires. The earliest recovery of the organism thus far is from the blood of a patient who became ill in 1947.

Evidence for Legionnaires' disease epidemics in America, some of which are still in progress, continues to accumulate, along with the knowledge that survivors of the disease may remain handicapped by it for years afterwards. A thirty-two-year-old Seattle woman, previously healthy and an avid skier, spent two months in the hospital beginning in February 1972 with what was later diagnosed as Legionnaires' disease. Seven years later, she still suffered repeated attacks of bronchitis and respiratory problems. About half of the Philadelphia victims had not completely recovered two years later. Permanent lung damage may result from the disease, and two women patients treated in Glasgow had long-term residual speech defects (ranging from five months to three years). Both women had virtually lost the power of speech for several weeks during the course of their illness.

Another thirty-nine cases of Legionnaires' disease arose between May 1977 and August 1978 among visitors to Bloomington, Indiana. Of these, thirty-five victims had spent at least one night at the massive "Stalin-Gothic" Memorial Union Building on the campus of Indiana University. Four of the cases were fatal. A new species of the Legion bacillus (now called *L. jordanis*), was isolated from four sites in or along the banks of the Jordan River or its tributary, which flows near the Union Building.

In August and September 1978, there was an outbreak of forty-four cases in the world's largest private hospital—Baptist Memorial Hospital in Memphis, Tennessee—that was ultimately traced to an auxiliary air-conditioning cooling tower that had not been used for two years until the pumps for the main cooling towers were inactivated by a flash flood on August 8. This auxiliary tower, unlike the others, had never had its water chemically treated, and there were two fresh-air intakes for the hospital just 50 feet away and 9 feet higher than the top of the auxiliary tower. The first case of Legionnaires' disease occurred three days after the auxiliary tower was put into service; the last case began nine days after the tower was again taken out of service.

Guinea pigs inoculated with water from this tower became ill with the guinea pig version of Legionnaires' disease. One still morning at 5:00 A.M., George Mallison, a CDC engineer with public health training, placed a smoke bomb in the cooling tower and watched intently as the smoke drifted from the cooling tower toward the hospital air intakes. The Legion bacilli apparently grew in the untreated water of the auxiliary tower (*L. pneumophila* grows symbiotically with blue-green algae that are often found in cooling tower water), and were then airborne in water droplets from the top of the tower into the nearby air intakes of the hospital. A column of mist rose some 30 feet into the air from this cooling tower (and from such towers generally), from which height microscopic flakes of algae and *Legionella* could drift over a vast area. Four of the Memphis victims had only walked in front of the hospital on the same side of the street as the auxiliary cooling tower.

It is less clear what happened in Philadelphia's Bellevue Stratford, although there is a cooling water exhaust vent just above the street where stood many of the victims of Legionnaires' disease. Whatever it was, it had happened before. After the Philadelphia epidemic of 1976, a member of the International Order of Odd Fellows (IOOF) recalled that a similar outbreak had occurred following the IOOF convention at the Bellevue the third week in September 1974. At least eleven Americans were ill; of fifty-one Canadians who responded to a questionnaire, a quarter had been ill shortly after the convention and one had died. Most of the victims had serum antibodies to *L. pneumophila*. Over half the employees of the Bellevue Stratford who had worked for the hotel for two years or more were later found to have antibodies against the agent of Legionnaires' disease.

The association of Legionnaires' disease with cooling water towers, suspected in Philadelphia, was proved in Memphis, and the point was soon driven home by events in Atlanta and Burlington, Vermont.

In July 1978 in Atlanta, eight cases of Legionnaires' disease broke out among golfers who played at a local country club. Investigation by the CDC epidemiologists showed that the vent from the evaporative condenser of the air-conditioning unit faced the tenth and sixteenth tees of the golf course, some 160 and 100 feet away, respectively. *L. pneumophila* was isolated from water in the condenser.

In Burlington, the results were much more serious. In April 1977 a thirty-year-old nurse in good health who worked at the 500-bed teaching hospital of the University of Vermont died of pneumonia. She had a mixed infection of *Legionella* and two other pneumonia-causing organisms. Because of the mixed infection, no particular emphasis was given to the presence of the Legion bacilli, which were already known to be widely distributed.

There was another case of Legionnaires' disease in a hospitalized person in May. In June, Burlington had three more cases of legionelliosis, out of which only one victim had been hospitalized throughout the normal maximum ten-day incubation period of the disease. But in July there were nine more cases, in August twelve, and in September twenty-eight. By late September, the CDC was asked to investigate, and a team under Claire Bloom, M.D., was sent to Vermont. Thereafter the epidemic dribbled off, with another thirteen cases up to the middle of December.

Reaction in Burlington to the epidemic was directed violently against the Medical Center Hospital. A typical comment was that of Jill Harris who, with her husband and a friend, owns a restaurant called The Snackery in a new shopping center overlooking Lake Champlain: "I wouldn't go there [the Medical Center Hospital], no matter what they say, and that's the way everybody I know feels about it, too...."[8]

The hospital was getting a bit of a bum rap, and not only from the citizens of Burlington. The lieutenant governor of Vermont, T. Garry Buckley, called on the State Health Department to restrict access to the hospital, while the Health Department was receiving some 40 calls a day from worried parents of the 15,000 students at the university.

Of the sixty-nine cases of Legionnaires' disease in Burlington that year, forty-one of the victims had been in the Medical Center Hospital for at least part of the disease's incubation period, but they had also spent at least part of the incubation period in the community as well. The other twenty-eight had not been in the Medical Center Hospital at all during the normal incubation period. Only thirteen of the victims had been hospitalized for ten days or more; these patients had most probably acquired the disease in the hospital. So, while it was clear that some people were contracting the disease in the hospital, others must have been exposed to another source or sources in the environs of Burlington.

Forty-nine of the sixty-nine victims of legionelliosis in Burlington were cigarette smokers; seven of the remaining twenty were ex-smokers. More than a third of those stricken were already so sick that their immunological defenses against infection were severely compromised and, naturally, those people had already been hospitalized at the time of exposure.

The initial American experiences with legionelliosis were with its epidemic form. But by the end of 1977, it was clear that sporadic cases occurred around the country as well. The results from Burlington made it clear that the disease was also endemic in some parts of the country. That is, a certain number of cases of the disease could be expected to appear in those regions year after year in the absence of an epidemic. Dr. Gregory Storch and his CDC colleagues studied serum from middle-aged and elderly Americans in four major cities.[9] They found that fewer than one in fifty of their subjects had antibody levels that suggested prior infection with *Legionella*. In endemic areas, the proportion of people with antibodies to the Legion bacillus was three to ten times higher.

Then Burlington, Vermont, had the dubious honor of being stricken by a second epidemic of Legionnaires' disease that was even worse than the first.

The CDC had been asked to investigate the first Burlington epidemic during the last week in September 1977, after fifty-four of the sixty-nine cases had already occurred. The EIS officers could find no common source for the epidemic. There were no further outbreaks in 1978, nor in the following year, and the staff of the Medical Center Hospital happily concluded that the 1977 epidemic had been a regrettable but transitory incident. Then, in May 1980, the disease struck again.

Two cases were harbingers of trouble. In mid-May, two maintenance men were working on a cooling tower on the Given Medical Building when they were accidentally sprayed with mist. Both workers became ill and, although both recovered, one was hospitalized with Legionnaires' disease for three months.

Linden Witherell, an EIS officer working as a local agent of the Environmental Protection Agency, had been worried about the source of Legionnaires' disease in Burlington since the first epidemic in the summer of 1971. After the Memphis outbreak, Witherell had asked George Mallison of the CDC whether the CDC could analyze water samples from Burlington cooling towers even though no epidemic was in progress. Mallison agreed to arrange the analysis, and Witherell, without much local support or enthusiasm, began to collect water samples from five of the city's cooling towers after the units were turned off in the fall of 1978. Analysis of the samples in Atlanta showed that only two towers were contaminated with the Legion bacillus. One was atop a medical center building known as the DeGoesbriand unit;

the other was the tower on the roof of the Given Medical Building. Both towers were cleaned according to the CDC recommendations in the spring of 1979 and were found to be free of bacteria. Strangely, the towers were neither sampled nor cleaned in the spring of 1980.

When more cases of Legionnaires' disease appeared in May, suitable steps were finally taken by the university's physical plant manager. The DeGoesbriand and Given Building towers were both sampled; chlorination of the water in both towers was begun on June 6 and continued for twenty days. The samples taken before chlorination showed that the DeGoesbriand tower was clean, while *Legionella* had reestablished itself in the Given Medical Building cooling tower, 600 feet south of the Medical Center's Mary Fletcher Hospital.

Chlorinated water is corrosive, and therefore chlorination cannot continue indefinitely. Following the procedure used by the CDC at the Memphis hospital, officials in Burlington used a biocide treatment with other chemicals to keep the cooling tower water free of algae and—they hoped—*Legionella*. The CDC experts were not invited to assist in the clean-up because Lloyd Novick, the Vermont health commissioner in Burlington, thought there was enough local talent to handle the situation.

There were more cases of legionelliosis in Burlington in July, after chlorination of the water in the Given Building had stopped, than there had been in May. Chlorination was begun again on July 17 and continued for the rest of the summer. By then, there had been eighty-eight cases of Legionnaires' disease in Burlington; nineteen were fatal. The victims' ages ranged upward from nineteen. One healthy thirty-year-old man who didn't smoke died even after being treated with erythromycin, which had proven to be the most effective agent against the disease.

Although the Given Medical Building tower was certainly the cause of many of the cases of Legionnaires' disease in Burlington, it was probably not the only cause. A sampling of the serum of some 600 Burlington citizens employed in various local industries (including the Medical Center Hospital) showed that 13 to 26 percent had antibodies against *Legionella*, indicating previous exposure to the disease.

By Christmas Eve of 1977, the status of Legionnaires' disease was very different from what it had been the year before. It could no longer be regarded as the cause of a single, bizarre incident. There had been 150 isolated cases scattered across the country, of which 32 were fatal; and four local epidemics had occurred in or near hospitals, which added an additional 91 cases and 23 deaths.

Besides the Vermont outbreak, there had been ten cases (one fatal) in and around Riverside Methodist Hospital in Columbus, Ohio, and to a lesser extent in a nearby university teaching hospital. Both hospitals had substantial construction projects under way during August 1977, when the epidemic occurred, and the Legion bacillus was later isolated from the cooling tower water of Methodist Hospital.

Holston Valley Community Hospital in Kingsport, Tennessee, in the southeastern corner of the state, had an outbreak of legionelliosis that more nearly resembled the one in Burlington, Vermont. There were thirty-three confirmed or highly presumptive cases of the disease, of which three were fatal. As usual, most of the victims (88 percent) were cigarette smokers. The hospital is located in a middle-class residential area of Kingsport. More than 5 percent of the residents of the area had antibody to *L. pneumophila*, a higher percentage than that found in either employees or patients of Holston Valley Hospital. Thus, Legionnaires' disease was endemic in the residential area surrounding the hospital (as well as in a similar control area in Bristol, Tennessee, some twenty-five miles east of Kingsport), but the source of the infections was never identified.

An epidemic of Legionnaires' disease that began in May 1977 at Wadsworth Veterans Hospital in Los Angeles has, like the Burlington, Vermont, outbreak, continued for several years; except that it is even more severe, with 199 cases through October 1980 (more than 30 of them fatal).

Wadsworth Medical Center's new six-story, $60 million hospital, set in a 600-acre parklike campus about halfway between Beverly Hills and the Pacific Ocean, and just off the San Diego Freeway, opened in March 1977. Two months later, the first case of legionelliosis appeared.

By Christmas Eve there had been nine cases; two were fatal. The *New York Times* quoted the hospital chief of staff, Dr. Earl Gordon, as saying that he did not consider that an outbreak or an epidemic of Legionnaires' disease was in progress at Wadsworth and therefore no special precautions were being taken.[10] Eleven months later, there had been forty-eight cases, of which sixteen were fatal. Kidney transplants had been suspended because six of the twelve patients given such transplants at Wadsworth in 1977 had contracted legionelliosis, one had died from it, and the "non-epidemic" showed no signs of slowing down.

Extensive excavation went on around the Wadsworth Medical Center in late 1977 as lawns and trees were planted, and CDC investigators isolated the Legion bacillus from a cooling water tower atop the Medical Center. By February 1978, the landscaping was completed, but there was no decline in the number of new cases. As soon as the organisms were discovered in the cooling tower water, chlorination was instituted until the bacterium could no longer be cultured from the cooling water. Yet the epidemic continued unabated. Half of the groundskeepers employed by the Medical Center had high levels of antibody to *Legionella*, as did about one in six (17 percent) of the hospital employees. Yet only 4 percent of the employees of a Veterans Administration Regional Office less than a third of a mile away and downwind from the Medical Center had significant antibody levels.

It may be that Legionnaires' disease is endemic at a low level in this part of Los Angeles. It is certain that most of the victims of the disease who had been employees or patients in the hospital acquired the disease in the Medical Center from some unknown source, since most of the victims had been in the hospital for seventeen days or longer before they became ill—longer than the incubation period. Even so, the chance of any individual patient acquiring legionelliosis in Wadsworth Medical Center was less than one in a hundred, although those whose immune response was impaired had a nine-fold greater risk. Unlike other outbreaks, cigarette smoking did not seem to be correlated with acquiring the disease in the Wadsworth hospital. Recently, by constant hyperchlorination of the drinking water and constant checking for the presence of *Legionella,* the Wadsworth outbreak has been reduced to a low level of new cases.

Not all of the more spectacular outbreaks of Legionnaires' disease took place in hospitals. On Wednesday afternoon, August 30, 1978, a Brooklyn physician, Dr. Ellie Goldstein, called John S. Marr, M.D., chief of the Preventive Medicine Department of the New York City Department of Health, to report that two brothers, aged twenty-six and twenty-nine years old, respectively, were in King's County Hospital with severe pneumonia and high fevers. Dr. Goldstein had worked at Wadsworth Medical Center and strongly suspected Legionnaires' disease. An older brother of the two sick men, Carlisle Leggette, had died in St. John's Episcopal Hospital six days before. When Dr. Goldstein learned of Carlisle's death, he had telephoned Dr. Felix Taubman, the director of the Department of Medicine at St. John's who suspected that Carlisle's death was due to Legionnaires' disease. After the two physicians compared notes, they had decided to contact Dr. Marr.

John Marr sent two sanitarians to the brothers' home in Bedford-Stuyvesant, and two epidemiologists to interview Joseph and Gilbert Leggette in the hospital. The preliminary investigation revealed that all three brothers had previously been in good health and that all three worked in New York City's garment district on West 35th Street, near such famous landmarks as Herald Square, Macy's, and the Empire State Building. Dr. Marr soon learned that the Legion bacillus had been isolated from Carlisle's lungs.

The investigation continued to center on the largely black residential area of Bedford until Friday of that week, when a call came from the CDC advising Dr. Marr of another probable case of Legionnaires' disease reported from Bellevue Hospital. The Bellevue patient lived in Harlem but worked on West 35th Street. As Dr. Marr explained, "That's when it clicked. We ruled out Bedford and concentrated on the garment district."[11] He immediately called the CDC and asked for an Epidemic Intelligence officer. It was 5:00 P.M., just before the Labor Day weekend.

Lester Cordes, M.D., from Atlanta joined the New York team over the weekend. Together, they looked over the garment district, although most of its businesses were locked up, and telephoned hospitals seeking additional cases. By early the following week the Bellevue victim had died and *Legionella* were seen in samples from his lungs. The Bellevue victim had been a "rack boy" whose job it was to push racks loaded with clothing from one establishment to another or between trucks parked in the narrow streets. Carlisle Leggette had also been a rack boy.

The garment district includes some sixty blocks of south-central Manhattan between Fifth and Tenth avenues and from West 30th to 38th streets. It provides employment for 75,000 people. News travels fast in the district—by the Tuesday afternoon after Labor Day, a local radio station got a tip that a mysterious disease had struck the area. Shortly after the broadcast, Dr. Marr's telephone began to ring. It rang incessantly throughout the rest of the afternoon, on into the evening, and beyond. It was ten o'clock at night before Dr. Marr could call Edward Koch and bring the mayor of New York City up to date on what was happening.

A hotline manned by forty physicians was set up to cope with incoming calls about Legionnaires' disease. It was soon logging 4,000 calls a day. Of these, nearly 200 callers reported symptoms suspicious enough to require further screening.

While the epidemic continued, Mayor Koch ordered his deputy director of operations, Paul Caswell, to coordinate efforts to combat the disease. Caswell promptly ordered all air-conditioning units in the garment district turned off. Water samples were collected from the cooling towers, and the towers were drained and refilled with heavily chlorinated water. Sanitation department trucks cruised the streets of the district spraying disinfectant. The subway entrances and platforms were also sprayed, debris was shoveled up, pools of stagnant water were removed, and everywhere wafted the scent of pine oil sprayed by the sanitarians to cover up the disinfectant odor.

Most employees of the district went on about their business, though much less confidently than usual. John Leggette, whose three brothers had all had the disease, went warily back to his own garment district job in early September. "I'm scared," he said, "but what can you do?"[12] John Leggette, like his dead brother Carlisle, worked in one of the offices of Interstate Dress Carriers, on West 35th Street between Seventh and Eighth avenues. Tony Thompson, who worked in a restaurant next to Interstate Dress Carriers, expressed a feeling of shock and powerlessness common to many of the district's employees. "It's like Jaws jumped out of the water and came to the garment district," he said.[13]

By September 11 the outbreak was over, at least for the time being. There had been thirty-eight confirmed, or highly presumptive, cases of Legionnaires' disease in the garment district, all of them concentrated in the single block between Broadway and Seventh Avenue (officially designated Fashion Avenue) and between West 35th and West 36th streets. Environmental samples of all kinds were sent to the CDC, but the CDC was buried in similar samples; it was not until December 15 that CDC epidemiologist Lester Cordes, by then back in Atlanta, called John Marr to give him the startling results.

The information that Dr. Cordes passed on to Dr. Marr on December 15 was that the Legion bacillus had been found in a cooling tower on the eleventh-floor roof of Macy's department store overlooking West 35th Street. John Marr transmitted this bit of data to the rest of the Health Department and to Peter J. Solomon, deputy mayor of New York for economic development. Mr. Solomon advised the health authorities to be "sensitive" to the impact that the news might have during the height of the Christmas shopping season, and it was a month before the New York City expert committee on Legionnaires' disease was told about Macy's cooling tower.[14] Of the thirty employees of the Interstate Dress Carriers office in the freight entrance of Macy's on West 35th Street, seventeen were ill, two had confirmed Legionnaires' disease, and nearly all the others had developed antibodies to *L. pneumophila*.

It is still not clear that Macy's cooling tower was the source of the epidemic. The organisms isolated were a different type (serogroup) of *Legionella* from those recovered from the two garment district workers who died, and samples had not been taken from the cooling tower until the epidemic was nearly over, so one type of *Legionella* could have been replaced by another in the interim.

If the source of the infection were a cooling tower, what then? There are approximately 9,000 cooling towers and evaporative condensers on Manhattan, all of which are potential homes for the Legion bacillus. Unfortunately, at this time, there is no generally satisfactory way of ensuring that the organism does not multiply in such towers.[15]

It is certain that Legionnaires' disease is endemic in the New York City garment district and elsewhere in the city. Later studies by the city Health Department and the CDC showed that 27 percent of workers in the district had high levels of antibody to *Legionella*, but so did people from other areas of Manhattan, as well as other parts of the city. At least one New Yorker in five has been exposed to Legionnaires' disease, making it the most heavily infected (hyperendemic) city so far discovered.

As the fifth anniversary of the 58th State Legion Convention in Philadelphia approached, a great deal of information had been amassed about the Legion bacillus, although many distressing questions remained unanswered.

Five hundred or more isolated cases of Legionnaires' disease are reported in the United States each year that are neither associated with an epidemic nor with an endemic center. These so-called sporadic cases are more numerous than those associated with outbreaks. In 1978–79, nearly 300 additional cases were associated with epidemics in a New York factory, a Wisconsin hotel (in which the organism came down a chimney and out through a fireplace into a meeting room), and in several hospitals other than those already discussed.

By June 1981, there had been outbreaks in California, Georgia, Tennessee, Indiana, Pennsylvania, New York, Vermont, Michigan, and Maryland (three of them before the Legionnaires' convention of 1976), and sporadic cases in Hawaii and the forty-eight contiguous states. Two states, Pennsylvania and Ohio, had more than 200 sporadic cases; Michigan, Connecticut, New Jersey, and Florida had between 100 and 200; and 5 other states (Iowa, Wisconsin, New York, California, and Massachusetts) had 74–96 cases. At the other end of the spectrum, New Mexico had had seven cases in five years, Montana two, and Wyoming and South Dakota one each.

One estimate put the annual number of hospital-acquired (nosocomial) *fatal* infections with *Legionella* at nearly 1,000; the estimated total number of cases of Legionnaires' disease in the United States each year is about 100,000.[16]

The organism had gone undetected for years because it

did not respond to the usual staining procedures for bacteria and because it was very hard to grow in the laboratory. There are still no staining methods specific for *Legionella* other than with fluorescent antibody, and diagnosis of legionelliosis is still difficult. The bacterium is widely distributed in soil and water around the world, and has been for years, if not for millennia. So far, although the organism can survive for months in tap water, its spread seems to be exclusively airborne.

The discovery of *Legionella pneumophila* cleared up the mystery surrounding a number of individual cases of pneumonia of unknown origin dating back to 1947. These investigations also showed that *Legionella* is a much more diverse species than had been originally thought. One organism, isolated from the blood of a pneumonia victim in 1947 and designated OLDA, an acronym derived from the name of the patient, is identical to *L. pneumophila*. Other previously unclassified organisms, similarly isolated from the blood or tissues of human pneumonia victims, have been collected in a new class called ALLO (atypical legionella-like organisms)—bacteria that have many features in common with *L. pneumophila* but are not identical to it or to each other. (This class of organisms is now called *Fluoribacter*.) The class of *Legionella* is also expanding. Besides the prototype organism, *L. pneumophila*, eight other strains of *Legionella* have been recognized by subtle differences in their metabolism and fluorescent properties, although all are capable of producing Legionnaires' disease (now better called legionelliosis). One of the newly discovered strains has been named *Legionella mcdadei* (more recently *Tatlockia mcdadei*) to honor Dr. Joseph McDade's epochal discovery.

Human red blood cells from different people, although nearly identical in every other way, may have different surface antigens, the well-known blood group substances A and B. This gives rise to four blood types, depending on whether the red cells have antigen A or B, both, or neither. Like the red blood cells of man, *Legionella pneumophila* was soon found to have different surface antigens, giving rise to what are called different serogroups. Thus, *L. pneumophila* exhibits eight serogroups based on different surface antigens. All are capable of producing life-threatening pneumonia in man and the number of known serogroups may increase with time.

Each year in the United States some 800,000 cases of pneumonia of unknown origin occur. The discovery of *Legionella* accounted for about 100,000 of these cases; the causes of the remaining 700,000 are yet to be discovered. So a great many other organisms capable of causing serious illness in man remain unidentified.

Legionella is ubiquitous. In some 200 samples from two dozen lakes in Georgia and South Carolina, 90 percent yielded *L. pneumophila*. It is apparent that *Legionella* and perhaps dozens of other organisms capable of causing pneumonia in man exist all over the world. Yet they remain unidentified because there has been, as one expert put it, "an almost complete cessation of inquiry into the basis, nature, validity, and limits of knowledge on infections."[17] It is a deficiency in our scientific efforts that is unlikely soon to be repaired.

And what of the unfortunate Bellevue Stratford, the "Grand Old Lady of Broad Street," where the fervor over Legionnaires' disease all began?

It did at least escape the fate that Philadelphia mayor Frank Rizzo had in mind for it. Mayor Rizzo wanted to demolish the beautiful old building and build a new one. Fortunately, a Philadelphia developer bought the hotel for $8.2 million, well under the asking price and less than it had cost George C. Boldt to build it in 1904. In due season the hotel was sold to the Fairmont chain of California and remodeled at the cost of some $20 million. Its capacity was reduced to 562 rooms, and, in late September 1979, the gleaming new interior of the Philadelphia Fairmont received its first guests. In September 1980, however, the original name was restored. Unfortunately, the towels, linen, and silver of the old hotel had been sold at auction, so all such appurtenances now bear the Fairmont label. But the "Grand Old Lady of Broad Street," once reviled and abandoned, has been restored to her former glory.

The dead Legionnaires, or those still bearing the scars of the disease, could not be so easily restored. There is still some bitterness among Legionnaires about the stigma that they feel the name of the disease has attached to their organization, and the tragic waste of life that accompanied it.

We now know that legionelliosis is a relatively common disease that has probably been killing people for centuries. Air-conditioning units are sometimes implicated in outbreaks, and nearby construction sometimes triggers epidemics. The 58th annual convention of Pennsylvania Legionnaires provided a cohort of victims of the disease that were linked by a common thread—attendance at the convention—and who were mostly state residents. Thus, their illnesses and deaths had an impact on state health officials that would never have occurred had the victims become ill in twos or threes in a dozen states, provinces, or countries, as had undoubtedly happened countless times before. The ordeal of the Pennsylvania Legion led to the discovery of legionelliosis and made possible diagnosis and effective treatment of the thousands of other cases of the disease that occur every year. With such proper diagnosis and treatment, the mortality rate for legionelliosis can be brought down from the 17 percent suffered by the Philadelphia victims to from 3 to 5 percent.

The veterans who died of Legion fever fell in humanity's longest and most bloody struggle, the never-ending war against infectious disease. That their deaths were tragic is indisputable, but they were neither wasted nor meaningless. In a very real sense they died that others might live.

The Center for Disease Control, for which 1976 had been a year of nightmare, had its tarnished image restored to its customary luster. As Dr. Edward Kass of Harvard

Medical School wrote in the *New England Journal of Medicine* in December 1977:

> These steps [the discovery of *Legionella* and the description of its properties], now recited as a brilliant example of scientific achievement, took six months and untold numbers of hours by large numbers of medical scientists with a variety of skills. Not long ago, such results might have taken years or decades. The understandable demand of the public and media for instant solutions to the problem should not be permitted to dim the magnitude of the present accomplishments. . . . This is a saga of medical science at its best, and the public have been the beneficiaries.

The Emperor's Sausage

"I would like to write a book about this experience. How it feels to come back after feeling that I was buried alive." Carolyn Wilson, forty-nine, was being interviewed by a reporter for the Albuquerque (New Mexico) *Journal.* It was no ordinary interview. Mrs. Wilson was in a hospital bed in the intensive-care unit of the Bernalillo County Medical Center, where she had been for nearly three months. Her husband, Warner, fifty-one, was also in the unit. Neither of the Wilsons could walk or speak. Carolyn's replies to the interviewer's questions were written out. Still, she could now open her eyes. When she was first stricken, "I didn't realize that the muscles in my eyelids were paralyzed. I just knew that everything went black, and I couldn't move. I wanted to scream, 'I'm not dead. I'm not dead!' You can hear everything all around you. Yet you can't move and you can't see."[1]

The Wilsons' terrifying experience began on Friday, April 14, 1978, in the east-central New Mexico city of Clovis, some ten miles from the Texas border. Clovis is a railway town, originally called "Riley's Switch." The tallest structure in Clovis is the grain elevator of the Curry County Grain Company that stands beside the Santa Fe railroad tracks. In 1907, the daughter of a Santa Fe railroad official was given the honor of renaming "Riley's Switch." She was studying French history at the time, so the story goes, and she was much taken with Clovis, king of the Franks, who converted to Christianity in A.D. 486.[2] In 1978, Clovis was a town of 40,000 persons, and neighbor to the Cannon Air Force Base, which was to play an important part in this story.

The previous evening Jonathan Mann, M.D., the young New Mexico state epidemiologist, was at home in Santa Fe preparing a talk for a health education class when the phone rang at 9:00 P.M. When an epidemiologist's phone rings, especially outside of normal working hours, it can mean a frantic journey to somewhere to deal with a sudden outbreak of human suffering, but the message brought by this call seemed fairly benign. It was the proverbial thin edge of the wedge.

The caller was Dr. Mitchell Cohen, a friend and former colleague of Mann's from the CDC. Mann and Cohen had been in the CDC's Epidemic Intelligence Service together.

Mitch Cohen passed on the information that a thirty-five-year-old enlisted man from Cannon Air Force Base had been flown to the William Beaumont Army Hospital in El Paso with a preliminary diagnosis of botulism. Jon Mann took careful notes as his friend gave the details of the case. Staff Sgt. Jimmy Bupp had become ill the preceding Monday, April 10, with a headache and extreme fatigue, followed by blurred vision and difficulty swallowing. Botulism frequently takes the form of a descending symmetrical paralysis that may begin at the eyes and end at the toes, and Bupp had the frightening feeling, common to botulism victims, that he might choke on every bite of food he ate. He had gone to the emergency room of the handsome USAF Medical Facility at Cannon AFB at 7:00 A.M. Monday, and he returned that evening at 6:00 P.M. He was then admitted to the hospital.

On Wednesday morning, Jimmy Bupp suddenly stopped breathing when his respiratory muscles became totally paralyzed. He was promptly put on a respirator following an emergency tracheostomy and flown to El Paso just before noon. Mitch Cohen knew that Bupp had been a part-time bartender at a Clovis restaurant, but he didn't know which one.

Dr. Mann thanked his colleague for the information, completed his notes, then called his assistant Dr. Ted Gardiner. Next he walked out the door of his home, east to the corner, and across the street. A few minutes later the two physicians were sitting in the Gardiner living room drinking coffee and organizing an investigation. Ted Gardiner called Dr. James Cook at William Beaumont Hospital, who was taking care of Jimmy Bupp. The diagnosis of botulism, as with many diseases, involves first ruling out other possibilities (stroke, Guillain-Barré syndrome, myasthenia gravis, poliomyelitis, other kinds of food poisoning, and so on. This had been carefully done. Mann and Gardiner would have liked to interview Bupp to learn what they could about where he might have contracted the disease. Although there are about ten outbreaks of botulism each year in the United States, most of them are small, involving fewer than three persons, and the vast majority (100 percent in 1979–80) are due to home-canned foods.

Bupp was on a respirator hooked up to the hole in his throat (tracheostomy) and couldn't talk. Ted Gardiner did the next best thing; he talked to Mrs. Bupp, who had taken a bus to El Paso to be with her husband. "No," she replied to his question, "no one else in the family was sick." Dr. Gardiner did learn that Jimmy Bupp worked as a bartender at one of Clovis's most exclusive eating places, the Colonial Park Country Club Restaurant, and this information was later passed on to Mitch Cohen at the CDC.

The next morning, Ted Gardiner drove to Clovis, where he was met by Jon Thompson, director of the state's Environmental Improvement Agency for eastern New Mexico. Gardiner was there to look for additional cases while Thompson and his staff inspected Jimmy Bupp's home and the Colonial Park Restaurant.

Ted Gardiner didn't find any more cases although Wilma Holland, a public health nurse with the state health division, called all the private physicians in the area seeking information about possible botulism victims. Jon Thompson, on the other hand, thought the problem was solved when he walked into the Bupps' little house at 116 Ventura and was proudly shown shelves groaning under rows of canned fruits and vegetables. But no one else in the family was ill. That didn't prove much since Jimmy Bupp ate mostly alone and when he felt like it. At the time he became ill, he had not shared a meal with his family for three days. His diet on the preceding Saturday consisted solely of popcorn and ice cream. Food samples from Bupp's van and from the refrigerator and his desk at Cannon AFB included kelp tablets, blackstrap molasses, and a lot of partly consumed and badly decomposed food.

As Jon Thompson said later, "By the end of the day we were supremely confident it was an isolated case of botulism."[3] To celebrate the rapid solution of the problem, Thompson and his wife went out to dinner and a dance that Friday night.

Some 200 miles away, in the state capital of Santa Fe, Dr. Jon Mann and his wife were having a small dinner party when Mitch Cohen called again from Atlanta about 11:00 P.M. Mountain Time. As soon as Jon Mann heard his friend's voice, he knew what had happened. "How many new cases?" he asked. "Two," Dr. Cohen answered.

Devota Martin had been hospitalized on Tuesday in Clovis. Then, on Friday, she had been taken to High Plains Baptist Hospital in Amarillo where Dr. Michael Ryan, a skilled neurologist, took over her care. That same Friday morning, Kathryn Bomar, a tiny, gray-haired, vivacious woman, nicknamed "Scoop" during her career as a newspaper reporter, had gotten out of bed and promptly fallen. Her left leg would not support her. Five hours later, Scoop Bomar was on her way to Amarillo's Dr. Ryan with a tentative diagnosis of stroke.

Although Devota Martin and Scoop Bomar had not known one another earlier, Mrs. Martin's son knew Mrs. Bomar's husband, Bill. The two men met again in the hospital corridor. The Bomars had eaten at the Colonial Park Country Club Restaurant on Wednesday. When he learned that Devota Martin had eaten there on Sunday, Bill Bomar thought that Dr. Ryan ought to know about it. He was right. Michael Ryan set aside his provisional diagnosis of "acute myasthenic syndrome" and called the CDC to report two cases of botulism.

Jon Mann brought the dinner party in Santa Fe to a speedy conclusion and, from 11:30 until 4:00 the next morning, was either on the telephone or conferring with Ted Gardiner. He and Dr. Gardiner flew to Clovis in a chartered plane early Saturday. They were met by an equally bleary-eyed Jon Thompson, who had been up most of the night reading about botulism.

By the time he met the plane from Santa Fe, Jon Thompson knew that the Roman emperor Leo VI had passed an edict in his capital (Byzantium) in the ninth century A.D. forbidding the consumption of blood sausage because so many of his citizens were dying mysteriously after consuming the uncooked meat. *Botulinum* is the Latin word for sausage and the modern name of the bacterium *Clostridium botulinum*, which produces the toxins that cause the symptoms of botulism, or sausage poisoning, as it was known until 1870. So prevalent was the disease a century ago that when challenged to a duel, the great German pathologist Rudolf Virchow (1821–1902) was said to have proposed sausages as a weapon.

Jon Thompson also learned that anyone eating any uncooked food probably consumes a few botulinum spores (the inactive form of the organism) without harm. Unless the spores germinate and begin actively growing and producing one of the eight botulinum toxins (each generally produced by a different strain of the bacterium, although some strains produce more than one toxin), they are completely harmless. Germination and toxin production requires warmth (usually), the absence of air and growth inhibitors, and a favorable level of acidity and nutrients. Even then, the toxins can be readily destroyed by heating food to the boiling point for ten minutes or to 180° F for thirty minutes. It is only when toxin-containing foods are eaten cold, or with inadequate heating, that poisoning results. Three of the eight botulism toxins do not produce disease in humans, Jon Thompson learned, and nearly 90 percent of human botulism is caused by either type A or type B toxins. So each of the trio that assembled on the Clovis runway that April Saturday knew the enemy. The problem was to find it.

At 8:00 A.M. there was a meeting with representatives of concerned groups at the Colonial Park Country Club Restaurant. The first decision was to close the restaurant. In response to the manager's anguished plea to be allowed to keep the bar open, Jon Thompson relented on the condition that no food of any sort be served. Martinis without olives and Old Fashioneds without orange slices became *de rigueur* at the Country Club bar.

The two physicians from Santa Fe set up a command post in the Environmental Improvement Agency office in the Bruce King Office Complex in downtown Clovis. By 9:00 A.M. Saturday, there were nine cases of suspected botulism—Carolyn and Warner Wilson had already been flown to Albuquerque for treatment in a chartered plane—and by noon there were ten more. It was a large and exceptionally severe outbreak. By early afternoon all the respirators at Clovis Memorial Hospital were in use and the situation was becoming desperate. It was saved by Air Force Maj. Joseph Begin, the hospital administrator from Cannon AFB who had been handling transportation problems. He arranged for a C-9 medical evacuation plane, called a Nightingale by the air force, to land at Cannon that afternoon.

At 4:30 P.M. a convoy of ambulances pulled away from Clovis Memorial Hospital and drove the half dozen miles to the air force base. Two minutes after they arrived, a DC-9 with hospital beds and a nursing staff dropped onto the runway and discharged its passengers, an air force epidemiology team consisting of Col. George Lathrup, Lt. Col. Patricia Moynahan, Capt. Royce Brockett, and Staff Sgt. David McClannahan, all of whom had come from the USAF School of Aerospace Medicine at Brooks AFB, Texas, to help with the botulism outbreak because of the involvement of air force personnel.

Soon seven botulism victims were carried aboard the aircraft on stretchers and four others walked up the ramp into the Med-Evac plane. Minutes later, the C-9 taxied past the rows of camouflaged F-111Ds sitting armed and ready alongside the runway; then, at a signal from the tower, it took off for Kirtland AFB in Albuquerque.

Bill Kinyon, a black-haired, athletic insurance man who was also president of the Clovis Chamber of Commerce, was one of those who walked aboard the Nightingale. As he later described it, "I woke up Saturday morning seeing double." He and more than sixty other prominent Clovis citizens had been at a banquet at the Colonial Park on Thursday night to promote a $2.4 million bond issue to support vocational education on the Clovis campus of Eastern New Mexico University. "I was trying some contacts . . . I thought it was those dumb lenses. I went to the optometrist but he couldn't explain it. Then my wife telephoned and said that there were four people in town with botulism. We took off for the hospital and they said, 'You've got it.' In the space of two hours there were eleven of us. . . ." Interviewed in the Bernalillo County Medical Center (BCMC) in Albuquerque, Bill Kinyon remembered his Chamber of Commerce duties: "Here we go to all this trouble to get Clovis on the map— but this is doing it the hard way."[4]

By midnight Saturday, Jon Mann and his team knew of twenty-six cases of botulism. Dr. Darryl Patrick of Cannon

AFB had provided half a dozen people who tried to call every one of the 800 persons who might have eaten at Colonial Park between Saturday April 8 and the following Friday. By late Saturday evening, the team had contacted 560 of the persons at risk. Dr. Mann had had a meeting with the Clovis City Council and the city manager and Ted Gardiner had called CDC-Atlanta Saturday morning to ask for 100 vials of trivalent botulinum antitoxin (effective against A, B, and E toxins). It was flown to Clovis and, by midnight Saturday, was being distributed around the Clovis area.

The role of botulinum antitoxin is to bind the toxin circulating in the blood and prevent it from reaching and paralyzing nerves. Thus the antitoxin must be given quickly while toxin is still circulating in the blood. It must also be the right type. Unfortunately, antitoxin is least effective against type A toxin, which has the highest affinity for nerves and quickly disappears from the blood. The Clovis toxin proved to be type A.

By midnight Saturday there were botulism patients from Clovis in BCMC and St. Joseph's Hospital in Albuquerque, in St. Vincent's Hospital in Santa Fe, at William Beaumont Hospital in El Paso, in High Plains Baptist Hospital in Amarillo, in Methodist Hospital in Lubbock, Texas, and in the Memorial Hospital in Clovis. Radio and television announcements alerted people throughout Texas, New Mexico, and Colorado to contact Clovis health officials if they had eaten at Colonial Park between April 9 and 14.

Jon Mann and his colleagues could do little more than send blood samples to the CDC laboratory in Atlanta, and further food samples to the FDA laboratory in Dallas, to be assayed for botulinum toxin, and then wait out the two- to three-day period before symptoms of botulism usually appeared. People sometimes become ill with botulism within two hours and symptoms are occasionally delayed for two weeks; but usually they appear within seventy-two hours of consuming food contaminated with the toxin. And, as Jon

Mann explained to reporters in a news conference the following Monday, they could reasonably expect 20 to 30 percent
fatalities in botulism victims. "What we fear is that the source
of the poison is a commercially sold food product, which
could mean others in all parts of the country will get a hold
of it also."[5]

A preliminary estimate of 800 persons potentially exposed included those who had taken part in a golf tourna-
ment at the Country Club and attendees at several banquets.
Equipped with membership and meal reservation lists from
the Country Club, a small army of investigators swarmed
over Clovis and its environs looking for more cases. It was
3:30 Sunday morning before Drs. Mann and Gardiner finally
got to bed; they were up again three hours later. If the Friday
meal at Colonial Park had also been contaminated, another
twenty or more cases of botulism might still appear. It was
for this reason that a second C-9 Nightingale was called in
from its home base in Illinois. It landed about dawn Sunday
morning.

The epidemiology team had tabulated the onset of the
thirty cases known by Sunday morning. Staff Sergeant Bupp
had been the first severe case (one in which the victim needed
a respirator to survive) the previous Monday. There were three
cases on Tuesday (two severe), another severe case on Wednesday, no cases on Thursday, eight on Friday (six severe),
then sixteen more on Saturday, although none of the Saturday
cases was severe. By Sunday, publicity about the outbreak was
widespread. Marci McSherry of the Poison Control Center
in Albuquerque was besieged with telephone calls and walk-in
inquiries from people who feared that their sudden attack of
abdominal cramps might be botulism.

The telephone interviews with possible victims continued
on Sunday. One interviewer called an Albuquerque woman
but was told by the woman's child that her mother was in
bed and very sick. An ambulance was called to take the woman
to BCMC, where botulism was diagnosed.[6] Sunday evening

the Clovis botulism outbreak made the national news on both CBS and NBC, and on Monday ABC had a camera crew in Clovis where Bill Redaker interviewed Dr. Jon Mann and a group of Clovis residents.

In the bed next to Bill Kinyon at Bernalillo County Medical Center was Clovis dentist Dr. Jacob Moberly. "I thought it was the flu," Dr. Moberly recalled. "Then my aunt came over and asked, 'Did you eat at the Club Thursday night?' My wife is on the board of regents at Eastern, that's why I was there. She ate too, but it hasn't bothered her. I had potato salad and she didn't, that's all I can think of." Moberly, like Bill Kinyon, refused a bed on the medical evacuation plane that brought him from Clovis to Albuquerque, but he got worse after the flight. His vision blurred and his speech became slow and thickened. His physicians explained that, although his blurred vision should clear up in three or four weeks, it could be six months before his speech returned to normal. He was understandably apprehensive about the future. "I have four girls; they'll just have to talk to my patients for me. . . ." Then, plaintively, "I hope people will understand."[7]

Although no new cases appeared on Sunday among people who had eaten at Colonial Park on Friday, three victims already in Clovis Memorial Hospital had to be airlifted to Methodist Hospital in Lubbock. The air force supplied ambulance service and a flight surgeon and flight nurse to accompany the patients.

Meanwhile, the total number of cases had risen to thirty-three. It was not the largest outbreak of botulism in the United States; that doubtful honor was accorded to the diners in a Mexican restaurant in Michigan where, in contravention of the law in Michigan (and in most other states), the proprietors served a hot sauce made from home-canned jalapeño peppers. The result was fifty-nine victims of botulism. Although the Michigan outbreak of 1977 was larger than the Clovis outbreak, it was far less severe. In the Michigan incident, only 6 percent of the victims required a respirator; in the Clovis case, 35 percent of those stricken required mechanical assistance to breathe.

In the first fifty years of this century, the mortality rate from botulism was as high as 71 percent. Only after portable respirators became widely available did it drop to the current level of 25 percent or less; but this still meant that eight or nine of the Clovis victims might die.

Monday, April 17, was relatively quiet. New Mexico's governor, Jerry Apodaca, was in Boston to compete in the Boston Marathon, but was being kept informed of events in Clovis.

By then it was clear that all the victims had eaten at the Colonial Park Country Club Restaurant either on Sunday April 9, or on the following Wednesday or Thursday, April 12 and 13. It was, unfortunately, far less clear what the toxin-containing agent had been.

Ironically, on April 12, there had been a "disaster drill' at Clovis Memorial Hospital in which smiling fourth graders were transported by ambulance to the hospital following an imaginary explosion at the school. All the while a very real disaster was gathering force in the community.

The FDA office in Dallas had been running so many botulism tests on mice with the food samples from the Clovis outbreak that they ran out of test animals and had to order an emergency shipment from Minnesota. The mouse assay, still the most sensitive and specific test available, involves injection into the mouse's abdominal cavity of half a milliliter of an extract of a suspected food (or the fluid portion of the blood of suspected victims). In from one to twenty-four hours, depending on the level of toxin in the injected material, the animal becomes excited, its fur ruffles, and its abdominal wall just below the chest begins to flutter. The wretched animal will ultimately die with typical symptoms of botulism if the dose of toxin is high enough. Other test animals receive the suspected toxin plus specific antitoxin (to type A, for example). The antitoxin that protects the mice identifies the type of toxin in the food or blood samples.

It was clear from the FDA results and those of the CDC that the Clovis victims had been poisoned by type A toxin. The only food sample containing toxin was a bit of potato salad from the Colonial Park salad bar. It had been prepared on Wednesday, April 12. At first blush, the problem seemed solved. The investigators remembered that Dr. Moberly was ill but his wife wasn't. He had eaten potato salad, she had not. The potato salad was contaminated. Ergo, it was the potato salad that was the principal source of the botulism outbreak in Clovis. But it wasn't.

In the first place, many of those who were ill claimed not to have eaten potato salad. Even more convincing was the fact that the restaurant's chef, David Natvik, told investigators that although potato salad was routinely made for the Club's Sunday noon buffet (and the first victims had eaten at the Club on Sunday, April 9), the leftover potato salad from that Sunday had been taken home by the restaurant dishwasher, Margaret Goodrich. Her family had eaten it and suffered no ill effects. This account was confirmed by Mrs. Goodrich herself. Moreover, unused potato salad was not usually kept for later use, and the leftover baked potatoes saved for the preparation of potato salad were always kept refrigerated until used. This was an important point. Spores of *C. botulinum* on the skin of potatoes survive baking, and the "heat shock" may cause them to germinate if leftover baked potatoes are kept at room temperature (as the events in a Denver restaurant later demonstrated).

Col. George Lathrup, M.D., Ph.D., and his epidemiological colleagues soon found that the only thing the victims of botulism had in common was that they had each eaten three-bean salad from the Colonial Park salad bar. This fit the distribution of cases on Sunday, Wednesday, and Thursday because the restaurant was closed on Monday and there was no salad bar on Tuesday. The question was, had three-bean salad prepared on Sunday morning been served again on Wednesday and Thursday, or had more than one batch of bean salad been contaminated?

The epidemiological results on the three-bean salad generated a new wave of excitement among the investigators. Find the three-bean salad, or the can(s) it came in, and any other cans of that brand still on the premises, and the problem may be solved.

It was Read brand three-bean salad made by Joan of Arc, Inc., an Illinois food producer incorporated in Delaware. Fifty-ounce cans of Read brand bean salad still on the restaurant shelves, along with an opened and partly empty can from the restaurant refrigerator, were shipped off to Dallas for testing. But of empty cans no trace could be found. Thus it was that, on a warm Wednesday morning, Drs. Mann and Gardiner, and Jon Thompson found themselves in white coveralls poised on the edge of the Clovis landfill. Their mission—to find an empty can of Read brand three-bean salad from the Colonial Park Restaurant.

It was easier said than done. The Clovis landfill was a great pit twice the length of a football field and nearly as wide. It was 30 feet deep at the deepest end; a three-story building would have fit in it nicely. The sanitation department had been told not to empty the dumpster that diners at the best tables in the Colonial Park Restaurant had such a fine view of. It was emptied anyway. The restaurant dumpster had also been emptied on Tuesday, April 11. This load contained the residues of the Sunday meal that had claimed the first five victims. Since then, sixteen garbage trucks had unloaded at the dump twice a day for a week. Looking for a needle in a haystack took on a whole new meaning to the reluctant trio of epidemiologists that sunny April morning.

It was not quite as hopeless as it seemed. The Colonial Park Country Club used garbage bags of a distinctive color and their garbage always contained the discarded boxes that golf clubs came in, so this "sentinel garbage" offered some clue as to where most profitably to search. Nevertheless, they examined the surface of the landfill thoroughly and found nothing. Then they called in a bulldozer and walked carefully through the new layer of trash that it turned up. But twenty-four man-hours of disagreeable work at the Clovis landfill failed to turn up a single empty can of Read's three-bean salad.

A couple of days later, Jon Mann told reporters: "It is becoming less likely that we will ever find the specific cause. . . . The clue to . . . the Clovis outbreak is buried under several layers of garbage. We may never know the ultimate cause."[8]

Further investigation revealed that the usual salad bar waitress was absent on Sunday, April 9, and that Staff Sgt. Jimmy Bupp, who had been demoted from his position as assistant night manager of the Colonial Park Restaurant to assistant night bartender, had prepared the three-bean salad that was the only food all the Clovis botulism victims remembered eating. Bupp took a bite of it himself, but "it tasted funny" so he didn't eat any more, but neither did he throw it away. The next day Bupp was the first victim of the Clovis disaster and spent the next four months in the hospital.

The standard procedure for preparing the three-bean salad was to open a 50-ounce can of Read three-bean salad (wax, green, and red kidney beans) and empty it into a serving bowl. A second can was drained free of juice before being added to the serving bowl. Jimmy Bupp did not drain the second batch, so his preparation of three-bean salad was particularly juicy.

For those whose knowledge of the Clovis outbreak came from television and newspapers, the episode was mostly all over. There was only one new case reported after April 17. But for others, particularly the victims and their families, the ordeal had just begun.

On Thursday, April 20, Randy Moore was released from the Clovis hospital, the first victim to be well enough to go home. By Monday, April 24, more than half the victims were out of the hospital, and the Colonial Park Country Club Restaurant was preparing to reopen the following day with an entirely new food supply. All the old stock had been impounded by the state. That same afternoon, the thirty-fourth and final case of botulism in the Clovis incident was reported in twenty-one-year-old Parker Miles, who had eaten leftover potato salad (and fed some to his Labrador) a week before. The dog was unfortunately diagnosed as having distemper and destroyed.

There was a first of a different sort two weeks later. John Garret, at sixty-five the oldest among the botulism victims and a pioneer Curry County rancher, died after a month in Methodist Hospital, Lubbock. He had been on a respirator all during his hospital stay and he developed a refractory respiratory infection that could not be controlled. At the time of his death, eight botulism victims were still hospitalized, seven of them on respirators. Among them were Carolyn and Warner Wilson, whose care was costing each of them $450 every day.

Frank Healy, the manager of the Colonial Park Country Club, estimated that it "may cost $500,000 to pay the medical expenses of the thirty-four victims." He went on to say that there was "no report of suits or contemplated suits."[9]

The first suit, for $750,000, was filed three weeks later. It was filed by attorneys for Howard Cowper, forty-nine, of Albuquerque, who was—unkindest cut of all—the executive vice-president of the New Mexico Restaurant Association, and who was still in BCMC. He had eaten at Colonial Park on April 13. The cause of his illness, according to the suit, "was the negligence of defendant and its employees in inspecting, preparing and serving to its patrons contaminated food." Cowper, the suit continued, "has suffered bodily harm, has required lengthy hospitalization, has incurred and will in the future continue to incur, substantial expenses for hospitalization and medical care. . . . Damages to cover cost of past and future medical care, lost earnings and impaired earning capacity and physical and mental pain and suffering."[10]

Three weeks later, Sandra K. Tybor filed a half-million-dollar suit against Colonial Park for her seventeen days in the hospital, and a week later Elizabeth Garret filed an $800,-000 suit for the "wrongful death" of her husband. In all, seventeen of the victims sued Colonial Park Country Club, Johnston Food Company of Amarillo, which had distributed the three-bean salad, and Joan of Arc, Inc., which had prepared it.

A visit of investigators to Joan of Arc's production plant in Chicago revealed it to be clean and orderly and the method of food preparation entirely sanitary. The company cooked the three-bean salad, which should have destroyed any toxin present; then the salad was acidified to a level that would have prevented the growth of C. botulinum. But it remained true that the epidemiological evidence pointed toward the Read brand bean salad as the culprit. The contamination in the potato salad, which was the only contamination actually found, was thought by the investigators to have arisen either because patrons used the same spoon for both salads (as they were frequently observed to do), or because juice from the three-bean salad dripped into the potato salad when the restaurant's patrons were dishing it up.

With the usual salad bar arrangement at Colonial Park, the potato salad was nearest the serving line, with the three-bean salad directly behind it. Jimmy Bupp's excessively juicy bean salad was particularly likely to have dripped into the potato salad, especially if the slotted spoon customarily used for serving the three-bean salad was exchanged for another.

Half the people who ate three-bean salad on Sunday, April 9, became ill, as did all those who ate the salad the following Wednesday, and nearly two thirds of those who ate it the next day. In contrast, of those who did not think they had eaten three-bean salad, none who ate at the Club on Sunday became ill, while 6 and 13 percent, respectively, of those who ate at Colonial Park on Wednesday or Thursday were affected, presumably by the potato salad. Only the three-bean salad was implicated statistically in illness contracted on Sunday.

Three-bean salad from Sunday may have been served again on Wednesday, though this is not certain. Salad served Wednesday night was almost certainly served again on Thursday. On Friday, April 14, three-bean salad from a new shipment was served and no botulism cases resulted among the diners at the Colonial Park Country Club Restaurant.

Five botulism cases resulted from the Sunday noon meal; four of the five were severe. Ten more cases arose on Wednesday, but only one was severe, suggesting that the toxin had been diluted. Of the nineteen cases that originated at the Thursday night banquet, six were severe, a higher proportion than for Wednesday, but much lower than for Sunday.[11]

It would be pleasing to combine these facts into a concise explanation of the origin of the Clovis botulism disaster. Unfortunately, no one has yet succeeded in doing so.

One plausible scenario requires that there were at least two contaminated cans of Read brand three-bean salad. The contents of the first were served on Sunday, April 9. On that occasion no contamination was transferred to the potato salad, perhaps because only ten people remembered eating bean salad Sunday noon. A second can of three-bean salad was opened Wednesday and added to the contaminated leftover salad from Sunday. The second can was not contaminated and thus diluted the toxin already present. On Wednesday the potato salad was also contaminated, probably by juice from the three-bean salad.

On Thursday, in anticipation of a capacity crowd, a third can of three-bean salad was opened, and this can also contained botulinum toxin.

This hypothesis assumes that the severity of poisoning of the victims is an index of the toxin level in the three-bean salad that they consumed. If, in fact, the severity of poisoning is a matter of individual variability, then a single contaminated can of three-bean salad explains the results perfectly well.

Some suspect that the contamination may have been deliberate. It has been suggested that Jimmy Bupp had a motive (resentment against the Club manager for his demotion); he had access to spoiled food, both home-canned and otherwise, and to the three-bean salad that he prepared at the restaurant Sunday forenoon. He could have deliberately contaminated that batch of salad; the toxin would then have been diluted by the addition of another can of bean salad Thursday night, and both the attack rate and the severity of the attacks would have decreased, as indeed they did.

So far, so good. But how to explain the increase in toxicity of the bean salad Thursday night (if there were any)? Bupp could have added beans, for example, contaminated both with toxin and with botulinum spores; germination of the spores, growth—and toxin production beginning after the Wednesday meal—would explain the higher toxicity of the three-bean salad Thursday night. But this explanation requires that the spores of *C. botulinum* germinate and grow not only in the refrigerator but at a level of acidity that the organisms tolerate poorly if at all. This proposal seems unreasonable, and so does the concept of deliberate contamination. Staff Sergeant Bupp, first of all, ate the contaminated salad and he became seriously ill. It's also difficult to imagine that he would know the ingredients he used in preparing the salad were contaminated and then taste the product. He denies any role in creation of the outbreak, and there is no reason to believe that he is not telling the truth.

Jimmy Bupp returned to Clovis to visit his former neighbors on his way to his new duty station at Edwards AFB in California, the landing site for the Space Shuttle, where he is finishing out his twenty years in the air force. The only apparent evidence of his illness is a very large, and very black, tracheostomy scar on his throat.

Colonial Park Country Club's own insurance companies —U.S. Fire Insurance Company of New York and Reliance Insurance Company of Pennsylvania—were also suing both Johnston Food Company and Joan of Arc, Inc. By the time the suits were consolidated and brought to trial, they totaled nearly $22 million, and Maxine Funkhauser, a former cocktail waitress at Colonial Park, had been awarded $11,400 in worker's compensation for the botulism she acquired while on duty.

In this century, there have been approximately a thousand deaths in the United States from botulism, most often from the consumption of home-canned foods. The common view that "sausage disease" is caused primarily by meat is not quite right; in the United States at least, most food-borne botulism results from vegetables, although in Europe the source is still most often meat. Recent culprits include corn, tomatoes, tomato juice, salmon, white fish, potatoes and peas, mixed vegetables, beets, figs, beef and mushrooms, mushrooms alone, carrots, chow-chow (a relish popular in the South, made with green tomatoes and peppers, cabbage, onions, red peppers, and spices), beans, mullet, applesauce, peppers, olives, and, in Alaska, seal and seal oil, muktuk (chunks of white whale meat with the skin and blubber), beaver tail, fermented salmon eggs, and fermented fish heads. A recent outbreak in Kenya was traced to the consumption of white ants (termites) kept too long in a plastic bag.

Commercial foods implicated in recent botulism outbreaks, besides the Clovis three-bean salad, include beef stew, tuna, chicken pot pie, cheese spread, Liederkranz, cherry peppers, mushrooms, and salmon. The outbreaks involving mushrooms and salmon led to the two largest recalls of canned foods in U.S. history; 75 million cans of mushrooms (in 1973–74), and 55 million 7¾-ounce cans of salmon (in the first four months of 1982). Of the millions of cans of recalled salmon (from eight of fifty-eight Alaskan canneries), only thirty have been found to be defective.[12] Food contaminated with either A or B toxins may smell and taste spoiled, but it should only be tasted after heating, as Jimmy Bupp can testify. Although the toxin type is not identified in more than half the outbreaks of botulism in the United

States, type A toxin accounts for most cases where the toxin is known, with types B and E a smaller number. In 1979–80, the ratios of A to B to E poisoning were 13:4:4.

Strains of *Clostridium botulinum* that produce type A toxin are most often found in the American West. The less discriminating B and E producers are willing to live elsewhere. Types C and D toxins are mostly responsible for outbreaks of botulism in animals (chickens, mink, horses, and cattle), most spectacularly in migrating birds, and sometimes in fish.

Botulinum toxins are generally absorbed from the upper small intestine, where they travel first to the lymph system, then into the blood, and finally to the junctions between the peripheral nerves (those not part of the brain or spinal cord) and the muscles they activate. If the toxin is present in sufficient amounts, the effect is akin to a scalpel stroke that severs the nerve—the muscle it activates becomes totally flaccid and remains so for weeks or months until the damage done to the nerve cell by the toxin can be repaired. What the damage is is unknown.

Botulinum toxin is one of the most potent poisons known. An ounce of botulinum toxin A or B is enough to kill about 30 million people—the combined populations of New York, Chicago, and Los Angeles. This extreme toxicity has another important consequence. So little is required to produce severe poisoning that the victim's body can't even make antibody against it, with the result that a person may be poisoned again by the same toxin since the first incident produces no immunity.

Part of the treatment of food-borne botulism involves administering the appropriate antitoxin. The only disadvantage is that this is made from horse blood and about one person in five reacts to the traces of horse protein in the antitoxin. Sensitivity to a severe reaction (anaphylactic shock) can be determined before the antitoxin is given. Although there is some argument about it, the administration of antitoxin to recently poisoned botulism victims seems to be helpful. Enemas and emptying and washing out the stomach (gastric lavage) also help to remove the toxin from the body. The enemas have a fringe benefit since botulism victims are often severely constipated by paralysis of their lower digestive tract. Aside from these measures and generally supportive therapy, there is little that can be done to alter the course of the poisoning, which usually results in a symmetrical descending paralysis. The more rapidly the symptoms appear after poisoning, the more serious is the outcome, as witness the cases of Jimmy Bupp and the Wilsons, all three of whom were acutely ill within hours of consuming the contaminated food and who were hospitalized for many months afterwards.

The Clovis outbreak was obviously one of food-borne botulism, which is what we generally think of in connection with this disease. Food-borne botulism is not an infection, since it does not result primarily from the ingestion of living organisms, but rather from the consumption of botulinum toxin. There are two other forms of botulism, however, both of which are the result of infection with living *C. botulinum*. These are wound botulism and infant botulism. Infant botulism may be the most common form of the disease, although it is the most recently recognized.

Wound botulism is rare. It results when botulinum spores germinate in a deep wound. Considering the ubiquity of botulinum spores, it's a little surprising that wound botulism isn't more common, but penetrating wounds are much more likely to be seriously infected with either of *C. botulinum's* close relatives, *Clostridium tetani*, the agent of tetanus, or *C. perfringens*, the organism largely responsible for gas gangrene (and a substantial amount of food poisoning). Recently, wound botulism was reported following the attempted intravenous injection of cocaine.[13]

It has long been medical dogma that botulinum spores do not germinate in the animal (human) gut and produce disease. It was never a very sound view, since there was evidence going back to 1922 that botulinum spores in animals could in fact germinate in the lower intestinal tract and produce toxin.

Then, beginning in February 1976, four California infants were diagnosed as having botulism. Two of the infants
had been primarily breast-fed, but all had some exposure to
other foods. A careful check revealed nothing unusual in the
diets of any of these children except that one had been fed
honey. Further investigation revealed that about one sample
of honey of every ten contained botulinum spores at levels
up to 70 spores per gram.[14] A tablespoon of such honey
would contain about 150 botulinum spores. The result was
that the Sioux Honey Association of Sioux City, Iowa (the
world's largest producer of honey), took the responsible step
of recommending that honey never be fed to children one
year old or less. This recommendation was endorsed by the
California Health Department and by the Center for Disease Control. It was an important warning because two major
textbooks on pediatrics, including one published in 1977,
recommend honey as an alternative to sugar or corn syrup for
formula preparation.

That honey frequently contains botulinum spores was
not particularly surprising; so do many other foods. It was
not long before an infant who had been entirely breast-fed
was diagnosed with botulism, although his mother's milk did
not contain botulinum spores. The conclusion was inescapable: botulinum spores (ubiquitously found in vacuum cleaner
dust, soil around house plants, and the soil surrounding victims homes) had been ingested by the infant even while
nursing at the breast, or while sucking his thumb or a pacifier.
Even this wasn't particularly surprising, as older infants, children, and adults are constantly exposed to botulinum spores.
But the second inescapable conclusion was that, unlike the
situation in people of other ages, botulinum spores were
germinating in the intestinal tracts of babies and producing
toxin.

Two years later, fifty-eight cases of infant botulism had
been identified in fifteen states and a case had been reported
from England. Since early 1976, more than 170 cases of
infant botulism have been reported, and we now know that

the earliest confirmed case occurred in 1931. Although cases have been found in Australia, Canada, Czechoslovakia, and the United Kingdom, the United States accounts for the vast majority of the cases reported thus far. Since *C. botulinum* is found in dust everywhere in the world, the disease is probably universal. The CDC estimates that up to 250 cases of infant botulism sufficiently severe to require hospitalization occur in the United States every year; an equal number of victims may be dying at home before signs of the disease become evident.[15] This combined total is some ten-fold higher than the number of food-borne botulism cases in the United States in an average year.

Ninety-eight percent of all recognized cases of infant botulism have occurred in babies between one and six months of age; the oldest was nine months, the youngest ten days; first-born children are infected less frequently than subsequent siblings.[16] Typically, the first symptom (often overlooked) is constipation, defined as three or more days without a bowel movement. Botulinum toxins paralyze the bowel and the bladder, and the child gradually ceases to excrete wastes. The result is a vicious circle. The constipation resulting from the botulinum toxin provides an increasingly rich and more extensive medium for the germination and growth of *C. botulinum* in the baby's gut. At one pole of response the baby suffers increasingly frequent bouts of constipation over a period of one or two weeks, during which time it becomes more and more inactive and weak. Its cry becomes increasingly feeble, as does its ability to suck or swallow. The eyelids droop, the pupils dilate and respond ever more sluggishly to light, and the baby becomes "floppy," especially losing the ability to control the position of its head, while its face becomes increasingly devoid of expression. Finally, the child may lie absolutely motionless in whatever position it is placed.

These changes are slow enough, and frightening enough to the parents so that most such children are seen by a physician and hospitalized if necessary. Severely affected babies, like other victims of botulism, frequently need mechanical assistance to go on breathing because of increasing paralysis of the respiratory muscles. Respirators are required in about one fourth of the cases of infants hospitalized with botulism.

As we have seen earlier, botulism can progress with frightening speed in adult victims, who may go from complete health to respiratory arrest within hours. In the United States every year more than 8,000 infants suffer what is called Sudden Infant Death Syndrome or SIDS (also called "crib death"). SIDS is apparently a complex of diseases that have in common just what the name implies, that otherwise healthy children die suddenly, most often while asleep. Some of these cases, although the percentage is not yet known, are the result of infant botulism in its precipitous or fulminating form. The age distribution of SIDS and of infant botulism is virtually identical. Neither occurs in the first two weeks of life and both are rare after seven months.

The toxins of infant botulism are the same as those of food-borne botulism, generally type A in the West and type B in the East, although a New Mexico baby from Acoma Pueblo was recently found to have type F toxin, and two of the first California babies with the disease excreted type B toxin.

No circulating toxin has ever been found in a child with infant botulism, so treatment with antitoxin is probably useless. Although C. botulinum is sensitive to common antimicrobial drugs like penicillin and tetracycline when tested in the laboratory, treatment with such agents seems to have little effect on a natural infection, probably because the concentration of the antimicrobials that can be achieved in the lower bowel is too low to be of much use. C. botulinum produces toxin in the late stages of growth, and the toxin is released when the bacterium dies and its cell wall disintegrates. An antimicrobial drug that killed C. botulinum in the lower bowel might cause the sudden release of overwhelming amounts of botulinum toxin, with a potentially fatal result.

Because infant botulism, unlike food-borne botulism, is an infection (with living organisms) rather than an intoxication (with ingested botulinum toxin), there are effective steps that can be taken to alter the course of the disease. Tube feeding of the infant, which bypasses the inability to swallow, causes intestinal movement (peristalsis) to begin again and empties the clogged lower bowel, thus reducing the level of *C. botulinum* and its toxins. This feeding can be made with expressed breast milk (milk removed by artificial means, such as a breast pump) for breast-fed infants to the benefit of both mother and child.

The mortality rate for the slow-onset form of infant botulism is less than 5 percent, while hospital stays vary from less than two weeks to more than two months. The baby gradually recovers perfect health even though it may go on excreting *C. botulinum* and its toxins for months. Why this is so is not clear. Probably the toxin ceases to be absorbed in the lower bowel as the infant's intestinal tract acquires its normal bacterial flora. Normal bowel organisms destroy botulinum toxin and prevent the growth of *C. botulinum* when they are cultured together in the laboratory and this phenomenon may play an important role in resistance to botulinum toxin.

What is it about the infant gut that makes it possible for *C. botulinum* spores to germinate, to grow so successfully, and to lead to the symptoms of botulism? Again, not all the answers are known. The question really has two parts: Why is the infant apparently protected during its first few weeks of life? And why is it protected after seven months but not between these intervals?

Dr. Stephan Arnon, the discoverer of infant botulism, and his colleagues in the California Department of Health Services have provided some interesting results (*The Journal of Pediatrics*, April 1982). They find that breast-fed infants appear to be more likely to have infant botulism than babies fed formula (possibly because mothers find it inconvenient to boil their breasts before nursing as they would a baby bottle and nipple). This might seem to be an argument against breast-feeding. The August 1982 edition of the *Harvard Medical School Health Letter*, however, repeats the earlier conclusion of the Committee on Nutrition of the American Academy of Pediatrics that "Breast feeding remains the best way to feed an infant." Breast-fed infants are statistically less likely to have the sudden-onset form of infant botulism that can be rapidly fatal. Infant botulism in breast-fed babies most often develops gradually. There may be factors in mother's milk (unsaturated fatty acids, for example) that inhibit germination of the botulinum spores. Babies fed entirely on formula are also protected from infant botulism for the first few weeks of life, although it remains a mystery why.

The infant newly delivered from its mother's womb has just come from an entirely sterile environment and its intestinal tract is also sterile. Immediately after birth, bacteria begin to colonize the bowel. The mixture of organisms found in the infant's bowel changes as its diet changes until, at some point, the baby has a population of bowel flora that does not permit the germination of *C. botulinum*. If this state is reached at about six months, it would explain the striking age distribution of infant botulism; but at the moment this is pure conjecture. Why do some infants get botulism while most do not? Again, genetic or anatomic factors may play a role, but what these factors are remains unknown.

Our story began with the events in Clovis, New Mexico, in April 1978. But even now the consequences of a few table-spoons of that fateful three-bean salad are still very much part of the lives of the surviving victims. Dr. Jon Mann and his colleagues interviewed the twenty-seven of the thirty-two survivors of the Clovis catastrophe who could be located at either nine or thirteen months after the outbreak and, two years after onset of the disease, sent detailed questionnaires to the same group, to which twenty-one responded.[17]

The group was divided into eight severe cases (those who had required respirators) and nineteen moderate cases.

The average victim of a moderate case of botulism spent about a week in the hospital, although one patient was hospitalized for seventeen days.

The victims of severe attacks of botulism were very much sicker and, in the Clovis outbreak, one patient in three was in this category. The severe cases averaged eleven weeks in the hospital with the bulk of this time spent on respirators. Both of the deaths from complications occurred in the severely affected group, and one of the severe cases was hospitalized for five and a half months.

Recovery from botulism, particularly the severe form, can be agonizingly slow. Of the eleven symptoms about which they were questioned, the average severely affected patient had more than nine at the beginning of his or her illness. Nine months later, the average "severe" patient still had more than six of the original symptoms, and two years later an average of five symptoms remained. This naturally led to severe depression and some of the victims sought psychiatric counseling. As one woman put it: "On discharge [from the hospital] the doctors told me it would be a few months before I was completely okay. After six months had passed and I was still not back to normal, I became very depressed. I can't help but wonder if I'll ever be able to perform as well as a woman of my age should."

Even symptoms that have completely disappeared under normal circumstances tend to return if the person becomes very tired. Kathryn "Scoop" Bomar, who was effectively blind for five weeks because she couldn't open her eyes, on a respirator for three months, and in the hospital for an additional month after that explains, "My voice still isn't back to normal and when I get tired my speech begins to slur and I have trouble making myself understood." For Scoop Bomar, it was six months after she left the hospital before she felt able to keep up with the housework and preparing meals in an approximately normal way.

Nine months after the outbreak, only one of the four severely ill patients who had a paying job before their illness had returned to regular employment. Carolyn Wilson, whose words began this chapter, remained on a respirator for a week more than four months, and in the hospital for an additional month. Her husband, Warner, had the unenviable distinction of being the most severely affected victim of the Clovis outbreak to survive. For an incredible five months and four days, he required the assistance of a mechanical respirator to breathe. The only bright spot was that he was able to leave the hospital ten days after finally being disconnected from the respirator.

Two years after the onset of illness, six of the seven severe cases who responded to the questionnaire reported that they still suffer from exercise intolerance. Of the six who had those symptoms in the beginning, five still suffer from general weakness, dry mouth, and shortness of breath, and about half still had shoulder/arm weakness.

The Clovis botulism disaster has no real villains; it is not a thalidomide story (see chapter 10). Joan of Arc, Inc., may have produced one or two cans of three-bean salad (out of many tens of thousands) that were contaminated with botulinum toxin, but the company showed none of the viciousness of Chemie Grünenthal or Distillers Ltd. that is described in the last chapter of this book.

Despite the severity of the outbreak, which might reasonably have led to the deaths of most, if not all, of those severely affected by the toxin, there were no deaths from botulism per se, but rather from the complications of long-term respirator therapy. The heroes of the Clovis outbreak are those who made this remarkable outcome possible. Perhaps the last word should be left to the air force epidemiologist, Col. George D. Lathrup, who concluded his report with these words: "This investigation was conducted under the supervision of Jonathan M. Mann, M.D. . . . of the New Mexico State Department of Health and Environment . . . [it] was an outstanding example of a fine cooperative effort by the civilian and military communities."[18]

A Virus of Love[1]

It began insignificantly enough on Tuesday night, four days after the TGIF party with her laboratory group. While showering before bed, Jeannine Karkasian, a computer programmer in her mid-twenties, noticed a persistent itching between her thighs. She scratched it enthusiastically with her washcloth and later with the edge of her powder puff.

The next morning she was very sore. The price you pay, Jeannine thought, for scratching too hard. On Thursday the pain was severe and radiated down both legs, but even with a mirror she could see only some diffuse inflammation and swelling. By noon, since she could neither sit nor walk comfortably, Jeannine went home to her apartment, made herself a very stiff drink, and climbed into bed after making an appointment at the employees' medical department for the next day. She was suffering from extreme pain on urinating and from overwhelming fatigue and intermittent nausea, very much as if she had the flu.

Friday morning, to her intense relief, she was much less miserable, but her nightgown was wet from a watery vaginal discharge. Even a casual examination revealed a ghastly change in her condition. Both her outer and inner labia on both sides of the vaginal entrance and beyond were marred with white, raised spots, some of them a quarter of an inch across, and with angry red borders. In all, she counted nearly two dozen of the ugly scabs.

Alternately frightened and angry, Jeannine bathed cautiously, dressed, and had a light breakfast before going to her appointment with a company physician.

Jeannine and some of her co-workers had gone out for drinks after work the preceding Friday. A few of them had gone on to dinner and dancing. One was a young man named Ted, a gangling Southerner with a delightful sense of humor. Both he and Jeannine were new to the group and they were immediately taken with one another. Ted ended up spending the night in her apartment. Jeannine, like the majority of contemporary American women, had been sexually active since her mid-teens, although she often went weeks or months without sex.

Ted had been a skilled and thoughtful lover and Jeannine had thoroughly enjoyed their lovemaking. But now she was angry and resentful. "I knew it must be something I'd caught from him," she told the physician later that morning. "He must have known he had it, but he didn't take any precautions to avoid infecting me. It's rotten that he's gone this week. I'd love to tell him what I think of him."

The doctor did a careful examination, took a blood sample and smears from the lesions with a moistened swab, then waited in her office while Jeannine dressed.

"I can't be absolutely certain until the cultures come back from the lab," she told Jeannine, "but I believe you've got genital herpes. Besides the external lesions, there are several in the vagina and on the cervix. If it's herpes, it'll clear up by itself in a few weeks. Meanwhile, I can give you something for the pain and antibiotics to prevent secondary bacterial or fungal infection."

"Will that cure me?"

The doctor shook her head. "Herpes is a virus and it's unaffected by antibiotics. All I can do is reduce the chance of secondary infections and try to keep you comfortable till the lesions heal. In a few weeks—it could be as long as six— they'll be gone and there'll be no scarring. They'll vanish without a trace."

"Six weeks!" Jeannine grimaced. "I hate having those things on me all that time. But if that's what it takes to get rid of it, I guess I don't have much choice. I suppose sex is out of the question?"

"Yes. You'd probably find it very uncomfortable and, at least for a while, there's a real chance of infecting your partner." The doctor paused for a moment. "There's another thing you should know. Genital herpes is incurable. The virus remains in your system forever and, at the moment, there's nothing we can do about it. There may be recurrences from time to time, as well. They can be frequent, years apart, or never. There's no way of knowing."

Jeannine was pale and trembling. "You mean I may go through this over and over and there's nothing I can do about it?" She clenched her fists. "That dirty bastard!"

The doctor smiled. "That's the bad news. It may come back. The good news is that it will probably never again be as bad as it is this time. Further episodes, if there are any, will be less painful and clear up more rapidly than now, and the lesions will probably be external. Nevertheless, I hope you'll come and see me whenever there's a recurrence so I can help you prevent complications. And you might send your male friend around as well." The doctor paused for a moment. "If you ever become pregnant, be sure to tell your doctor that you've had genital herpes. It's very important."

Jeannine Karkasian, a slender, dark-haired woman, is attractive and vivacious. She easily draws men's attention. But her infection with genital herpes completely altered her self-image for a long time. She thought of herself as ugly and diseased, worse still, infectious. Jeannine's love affairs had usually been long-term relationships in which sex played an important part. Now she feared that she could never again have such intimacy because she would ultimately infect her partner.

Then she read an article in a woman's magazine about genital herpes that stressed the link between such infection and the subsequent risk of cervical cancer. The article also mentioned that a majority of infants infected with herpes during delivery either die or have serious birth defects. She reacted to the article with shock and horror. Her brief encounter with Ted had left Jeannine a sick and frightened young woman. In fact, because of its recurrence and incurability, genital herpes has a more devastating emotional impact on couples, and particularly on women, than does gonorrhea. It has driven some victims to suicide.

Jeannine Karkasian is not her name, but her experience is real. Genital herpes is not a reportable disease, so figures on its incidence are educated guesses supplemented by information on the numbers of people who have antibodies to the virus in their blood. At least 300,000 new cases of genital herpes appear each year in the United States. The total number of people who have had prior exposure to herpes virus is perhaps 50 or more million, of which as many as one third have had genital herpes. The majority of this vast number of people don't even know they've had the disease, and there are a small number of people who do not form antibodies to the organism even a year after the virus has been isolated from them.

In herpes or VD clinics, the average age of women appearing with genital herpes is between twenty-two and twenty-six, with men averaging a few years older. For both sexes the majority have had only one sex partner in the three or so months before appearance at the clinic, although the range is typically one to seven, with little difference between men and women.[2]

The lesions of an initial infection in women last slightly more than two weeks on the average. Pain in varying degrees is present most of that time. It is severe for the first week or so, then moderate for a few days, and mild thereafter. The lesions in either sex, whether initial or recurrent, resemble second-degree burns and may feel like them. One young man graphically described it as feeling as if a hot soldering iron was being held against his penis.

A woman is capable of transmitting her infection (that is, she is shedding infectious virus) for about nine days of the sixteen that the lesions typically last. In nearly nine of every ten initial infections, the uterine cervix also has herpes-infected lesions.

In recurrences, the periods of pain and of virus shedding are only about half as long as in the original infection, and the lesions last an average of ten rather than sixteen days. The pain associated with recurrences is usually mild and there are only half as many lesions as in the initial infection (an average in recurrences of about half a dozen in both men and women, although many victims may have only one or two). In recurrences, cervical lesions appear in only about one out of ten patients.

In men, the lesions on the penis caused by initial infection last about three days longer than in women, and shed virus longer, but they remain painful for only about ten days compared with more than two weeks in women. Recurrences in men are much less distressing than the initial infection. The lesions may last ten days, instead of two and a half weeks, but they shed virus for less than four, and are painful for only two or three days.

The earliest lesion of genital herpes on dry skin like the outer labia, thighs, buttocks, or the shaft of the penis is a fluid-filled vesicle that later ruptures to form a shallow ulcer that may resemble the ulcers of syphilis. The ulcer quickly scabs over and subsequently heals. In moist locations like the inner labia or under the foreskin of uncircumsized men, vesicles seldom form; the initial lesion is the ulcer. The ulcers, wherever they're found, are obviously susceptible to bacterial and yeast infections.

Recurrences in both sexes vary wildly in frequency. One woman with recurrent genital herpes had a recurrence with ulcerated lesions that healed within four days of their initial appearance. Eight days later, she had another episode that lasted three days. And three days after those lesions had healed, she had another brief recurrence. In other cases, the interval between recurrences may be months or years, or the disease may never reappear. In one group of twenty-six women attending a genital herpes clinic, three had recurrences once a year, seven had lesions every three to six months, and sixteen had recurrences every two months or more often.[3] The frequency of recurrences diminishes sharply after the first two years, and approximately one out of three victims of known genital herpes never has a recurrence. Women generally have fewer recurrences than do men.

A recent study of some 3,100 middle- to high-economic-level men and women (*Sexually Transmitted Diseases*, January–March 1982) found, however, that over two thirds of the subjects had more than five relapses a year, with a nearly equal rate for both sexes. Nearly a quarter had recurrences every month and these recurrences were more painful for women, and the frequency of recurrence did not diminish with time.

Unfortunately, both men and women may be initially and recurrently infected and infectious without showing any symptoms. This may be true of half the initial infections and a much higher proportion of recurrences. Fortunately, the amount of virus shed in the absence of lesions is small. Nevertheless, this makes foolproof avoidance of infection impossible by any means less drastic than strict fidelity to one uninfected partner—or complete abstinence. Even this may not be enough if recent results from UCLA prove to be correct. According to a brief article in the July 1982 issue of *Discover*, California scientists have found that herpes simplex virus can survive for three days in gauze, for eighteen hours on medical instruments, and—perhaps most important—for four hours on toilet seats. It is not yet clear that the organisms remain infectious under these conditions, but the implications are worrisome.

Genital herpes is caused by herpes simplex virus, type 2, or HSV-2, for short. It is a tiny organism. If all 8 million inhabitants of New York City were shrunk to the size of herpes viruses—an appealing idea in many ways—then lined up side by side, they would barely extend across the word "Manhattan." As a practical matter, the virus is smaller than the pores in a condom, so this form of protection isn't much good.[4]

In all, there are some fifty known herpes viruses infecting thirty species of animals, including frogs, snakes, sharks, and oysters, but only five affect man. Most of us have been exposed to at least three of the five and have antibodies to prove it.

One herpes virus (called VZ) causes chicken pox (varicella) in children and recurs as shingles (herpes zoster) in adults. Another (the Epstein-Barr virus) causes infectious mononucleosis and a type of human cancer called Burkitt's lymphoma, which is common in parts of Africa. A third member of the group (cytomegalovirus, or salivary gland virus) causes an often fatal illness in newborns. Herpes simplex virus also causes the familiar cold sores around the mouth. Most adults have antibodies to at least one of the herpes simplex viruses, to varicella–herpes zoster, and to cytomegalovirus.

Tiberius, Roman emperor at the time of Christ's death, once banned kissing in public places in an effort to stop the spread of cold sores. It was not until the 1950s, when isolation and identification of viruses became possible, that it became clear that the herpes simplex virus that caused cold sores was usually acquired in childhood and then reappeared from its latent state in the human body upon suitable provocation (fatigue, tension, cold, or sunlight, among other factors). It was 1967 when virologist Dr. Walter Dowdle at the Center for Disease Control (where he now heads the Center for Infectious Disease), and his colleagues showed that herpes simplex virus exists in two distinct forms, HSV-1 and HSV-2. Dowdle and his co-workers also found that HSV-2 predominated in genital herpes, while HSV-1 was the form of the virus found in cold sores and other "above the waist" herpes infections.

The author of a highly regarded textbook on diseases of the vulva published in 1954 said that she had never seen a case of genital herpes in her practice. More than ten years later, an equally prominent gynecologist said that he had seen only two or three cases in his career.[5] Since then the disease, for whatever reason, has become much more widespread. In the CDC's view, an epidemic of genital herpes began in 1966; over the next thirteen years, the rate at which patients consulted private physicians for genital herpes infection increased nearly nine-fold.[6] The idea that genital herpes is caused only by HSV-2 while oral herpes is caused only by HSV-1 is increasingly less accurate and on the road to becoming useless.

In one recent investigation, typing of the herpes virus involved in 100 genital infections yielded 81 of the "genital" strain of herpes, HSV-2, and 19 of the "oral" strain, HSV-1. Herpes infections around the mouth may also be caused by HSV-2, the "genital" strain. Some of this scrambling of "site-specific" strains results from self-infection. Virus can be transferred on the fingers from the lips to the genitals, or vice versa. Occasionally the fingers can also become painfully infected with either type 1 or type 2 viruses, if there is a break in the skin through which the virus can enter. Prior infection with HSV-1 does lead to milder cases of genital herpes because antibodies to HSV-1 react to some extent with HSV-2.

Auto-inoculation, as it is also called, is generally involved in oral-genital infections in small children where the same virus type is found in both locations. The major contributor to HSV-1 appearing as a genital infection, however, or of HSV-2 appearing around the mouth, is direct oral-genital contact, and this appears to be a phenomenon of increasing popularity, especially among the young. Genital infection with HSV-1, although as initially unpleasant as the similar infection with HSV-2, has far less tendency to recur.

Antibodies to HSV-2 are virtually unknown in nuns and nearly universal in prostitutes—strong evidence for regarding genital herpes as a venereal disease—and HSV-2 has also been transmitted by sexual contact in several species of experimental animals. There are a few cases of transfer of herpes virus via eating utensils, cups, and the like.

According to some estimates, about one third of the population of the United States age thirty-five or older has antibodies to HSV-2, and at least twice that many have antibodies to HSV-1. The presence of antibody is related to socioeconomic status (SES). A third to a half of adults in high SES groups have HSV antibodies, while 80 to 100 percent of those in low SES groups have such antibodies. Antibodies to HSV-2 are seen in only about 10 percent of high SES adults, but in two to six times as many low SES adults. In the course of a year, an estimated 15 million Americans will have two or more recurrences of oral or genital herpes. But what happens to the virus between such flare-ups?

The organism takes its name from the Greek verb *herpein* —to creep—and, although this is not the origin of the name, the answer to the question of its location between recurrences is that the virus moves slowly (about 1 inch in sixteen hours) along the nerve fibers until it arrives either at the lumbrosacral ganglion* in the pelvis near the base of the spine, or at the trigeminal ganglion of the fifth cranial nerve at the base of the brain near the cheekbone, depending on where it started.

In either location it waits—as intact virus or viral subunits—until some stimulus like fatigue, illness, or stress causes

---

* A ganglion is, literally, a swelling at the branch points of nerves.

it to begin its leisurely journey back toward the lips or the genitals. HSV-1 can be found on autopsy in both the left and right trigeminal ganglia in about half the bodies examined. An alternative theory is that the virus particles continually move between nerve and skin but that the immune system is usually healthy enough to eliminate them before they cause skin eruptions.

Most of the time, the virus in the trigeminal ganglia retraces its steps to the lips whence it came. Occasionally, it takes a far more dangerous path that fans out over the base of the brain and can lead to herpes encephalitis, a disease that, untreated kills seven of every ten victims. This condition is not rare. It is the most common cause of fatal encephalitis not due to an external agent. Many victims of herpes encephalitis are diagnosed as having a psychiatric disorder; conclusive diagnosis requires a brain biopsy. Of survivors of untreated herpes encephalitis, fewer than one in ten recover complete brain function.[7] According to a report in the *Journal of Infectious Diseases* for June 1982, of 106 brain biopsy samples, 102 were HSV-1; apparently HSV-2 plays a minor role in this disease. Primary infection appeared most often in the young (average age, eighteen years) while those with recurrent herpes infection leading to encephalitis averaged forty-six years of age.

As one pair of authors on herpes encephalitis wrote: "It is disquieting to recognize that in the vast majority of us a lethal encephalitis virus lies latent within millimeters of the brain. . . ."[8] They go on to point out that perhaps a cold sore, annoying though it may be, should be welcomed as evidence that the virus has taken its usual benign course rather than spreading upward into the brain.

Fortunately, herpes encephalitis is now potentially treatable, as we'll see later, though it remains a very serious disease in which about a third of its victims die despite treatment and the proportion of brain-damaged survivors is high. Estimates of the incidence of herpes encephalitis vary from a few hundred to a few thousand each year in the United States.

Recurrent herpes is unpleasant enough; but some of its complications, such as herpes encephalitis, are far worse. Herpes keratitis, which results from the virus multiplying in and around the eye after being transferred from a lesion on the lips or the genitals, is the leading infectious cause of blindness, and is responsible for between 10,000 and 20,000 cases each year.

Of particular interest to women are the two much discussed herpes complications—cervical cancer and infants infected in the womb or at birth.

If a woman has a recurrence of active genital herpes at the time her baby is delivered, the child can be infected during passage through the birth canal. A recurrent infection, if it is confined to the cervix or vagina, may be unnoticed by the expectant mother. The result of such infection of a child during or before delivery is appalling, and the chance that a mother with active genital herpes will infect her child is about 50:50. About two thirds of babies so infected die within a week of birth, and at least half of the survivors are severely defective, usually because of failure of the head and brain to continue development (microcephaly). Three fourths of infants with herpes have HSV-2; the remainder have HSV-1.

In the event that an expectant mother has a flare-up of genital herpes about the time she is expected to deliver, the safest procedure is to have a Caesarean section. This should be done before the fetal membranes rupture because newborns have been infected with genital herpes when left in the womb for several hours after the loss of the protective membranes. Initial infections with genital herpes are particularly dangerous to the baby, perhaps because of the high level of virus shed in such infections. Unfortunately, 70 percent of women who deliver babies with HSV infections have no sign of the disease within eight weeks of delivery.

Herpes infections in newborns are usually recognized by the appearance of typical herpes lesions of the eye, skin, or mouth. As Dr. Ann Arvin and her colleagues in San Francisco point out (*Journal of Pediatrics*, May 1982), however, only about one third of newborns with widespread (disseminated) herpes or herpes encephalitis have such lesions. The results are tragic. In the California study, five of six children with disseminated herpes died within twelve days. The only survivor received early antiviral therapy. This infant was delivered by Caesarean section from a mother with active genital herpes more than twenty-four hours after the fetal membranes had ruptured. Of eight newborns with herpes encephalitis, five died at intervals up to half a year; the three survivors were severely brain-damaged (blind, spastic, and severely microcephalic).

Herpes infection of a newborn baby is a frightening prospect, but in fact the risk is very low. Considering the incidence of genital herpes, infant herpes is an astonishingly rare disease—perhaps because the mother's resistance to herpes recurrence seems to increase toward the end of her pregnancy. Infant herpes was estimated to occur in between 100 and 1,000 infants in 1979.[9] This is out of some 3.5 million births, of which at least 500,000 must have been to women with antibodies to HSV-2.

Not all women plan to have children. But all women who still have a uterus are concerned about the risk of cervical cancer. The risk of developing cervical cancer is five to eight times higher in women who have genital herpes. This is a fact worth examining in some detail.

We have seen that herpes infection of the cervix is very common in initial genital herpes infections and in about one in ten recurrences. Herpes simplex viruses cause cancer when injected into some experimental animals. Do they cause cancer of the cervix in humans?

The epidemiological evidence says yes. In the opinion of some investigators, this evidence is as good as the data that originally linked cigarette smoking with lung cancer. As I've pointed out before, most scientists agree that epidemiological evidence never proves anything, it can only indicate factors that need investigation. In the case of the link between cigarette smoking and lung cancer, the evidence is now so overwhelming that it's difficult to find a scientist not employed by the Tobacco Research Institute who questions the data. The connection between cervical cancer and genital herpes is not nearly so clear-cut.

Something like one woman in three has antibodies to HSV-2, indicating a previous infection with the virus, whether apparent or otherwise. Yet a much smaller proportion of women ever develop cervical cancer. So it is clear that the mere presence of the virus is not a sufficient condition for development of a malignancy. Something else is involved.

What that something else might be is suggested by the work of Dr. Laure Aurelian of Johns Hopkins University School of Medicine (to whom I helped teach biochemistry when she was a medical student) and her colleagues. The important conclusion from their work was contained in a *Science* article that the Hopkins group published in 1973.[10] As reported in this paper, they measured antibody to a crude surface antigen of HSV-2–infected cells in the blood of women with atypical cells from a Pap smear (a premalignant condition), in women with *in situ*, or localized, cancer of the cervix, and finally in women with invasive cancer originating from the cervix.

The mean age of those women with atypical cells in their Pap smears was thirty-four. Of those with carcinoma *in situ* the mean age was thirty-nine, while that of women with invasive cancer was fifty-two. Thus, there was an interval of some eighteen years in this population of patients from the first appearance of atypical cells to the development of virtually incurable cancer. These data point up the great utility of regular Pap smears and the slowness with which cervical cancer develops. The main point of the paper, however, lay elsewhere.

The data of Aurelian and her colleagues showed that only 35 percent of the women with atypical cervical cells had antibody to the crude surface antigen called HG-4, while none of the normal controls did. With carcinoma *in situ*, the percentage of women with antibody to HG-4 rose to 68 percent

(5 percent of the controls had the antibody), and, of those women with invasive cancer, 91 percent had antibody to HG-4, while only 10 percent of the controls did. The controls were matched for age, race, and socioeconomic status. So perhaps the ability to form antibody to HG-4 (and another antigen from herpes-infected cells called AG_e) is related to susceptibility to cervical cancer.

This work is being pursued by Dr. Aurelian and her colleagues at Hopkins, and at other laboratories around the world. But whether HSV-2 *causes* cervical cancer remains to be proved. Certainly a prudent woman who knows that she has had genital herpes should have a Pap smear at least once a year and possibly oftener.

It has also been proposed that multiple sclerosis is caused by HSV-2 in a small number of people who lack antibodies to HSV-1. This intriguing hypothesis of Dr. John Martin of the National Institutes of Health in Bethesda, Maryland, rests on a considerable amount of epidemiological evidence.[11]

The herpes viruses, like other viruses, are intracellular parasites incapable of independent growth. They invade body cells and commandeer the cell's metabolic machinery, shutting off synthesis of normal cellular DNA, RNA, and protein, and reprogramming the cell to make only the materials necessary for the production of new virus particles. A single virus can appropriate the metabolic equipment of a normal cell and use it to make tens of thousands of copies of the infecting virus, which then, in the case of herpes, leak from the cell to attack other cells and leave behind the burned-out hulk of a virus factory.

Because the viruses can pass from cell to cell without entering the extracellular fluid, they are difficult to attack with drugs. The problem is made more difficult by the fact that the virus particles have virtually no independent metabolism of their own.

Some herpes victims have spent thousands of dollars on "cures" for the disease. The "cures" all seem to work, because the disease is self-limiting and will go away in time whether the lesions are smeared with Skippy peanut butter, diesel fuel, or holy water. The trick is to prevent recurrences and to reduce pain and the production of new lesions. Since recurrence tends to diminish with time, all remedies seem to work here too, if they are only adhered to long enough. The situation is ideal for quackery, and quacks have taken full advantage of it to fatten on the fears of the gullible and desperate.

Lupidon G vaccine is a heat-inactivated strain of HSV-2. It and vaccines for other diseases (for example, smallpox and yellow fever) that have been used to treat herpes are ineffective against herpes; furthermore, like all vaccines, there is some risk associated with their use. Specific diets or dietary supplements (vitamins, zinc, lysine) are useless, as are a variety of substances (ether, Betadine, silver sulfadiazine, the spermicide Nonoxynol-9, steroid creams, and dimethylsulfoxide or DMSO) applied directly to the lesions. The metabolic inhibitor 2-deoxy-D-glucose is ineffective (*Journal of Infectious Diseases*, August 1982) and potentially dangerous.

There are, however, experimental drugs that show great promise in treating herpes, particularly the life-threatening herpes encephalitis, and herpes keratitis, which can cause blindness. Fortunately, herpes virus is relatively unusual among viruses in forcing the cells it invades to make some enzymes needed for viral replication that are unique to the virus. Since these herpes enzymes are different from those in the host cell and are essential for viral replication, they offer a potentially useful point of attack for stopping the viral infection.

Ideally, such a drug should abort a recurrent viral infection when given to a patient who was suffering the localized pain and itching that often signals an imminent recurrence. Likewise, given early in infection, the drug should stop the production of new vesicles or ulcers and promote the rapid healing of those already formed. Most important of all, a successful drug should stop the sinister progress of herpes encephalitis and the ravages of herpes keratitis. Finally, such a therapeutic agent should be reasonably free of dangerous or excessively unpleasant side effects, it should not promote or induce cancer or birth defects in experimental animals, and it should be useful for local application to the skin or eyes and for injection. Needless to say, no such drug exists.

The search for such wonderful compounds has been under way for decades in many laboratories, and, fortunately, animal models for genital herpes exist (female mice and guinea pigs). Recently, this extraordinary effort seems to be bearing fruit, which is important not only for the millions of sufferers from the usual herpes infections (to say nothing of other viral maladies), but for cancer and organ transplant patients whose natural immunity has been suppressed by drugs as part of their treatment. More than 70 percent of all cancer and transplant patients have painful and sometimes fatal herpes infections.

There is now a drug, 5-iododeoxyuridine, or IDU, that is effective against herpes keratitis. Unfortunately, it has too many undesirable side effects to be injected, and it is useless against the skin lesions of herpes. Another drug, adenosine arabinoside, or ara-A (Vidarabine) is effective when given by injection for treating herpes encephalitis, although it is relatively insoluble in body fluids and, once dissolved, is quickly broken down in the body so that large doses must be given. It must also be given early in the infection—when accurate diagnosis is difficult. Without early treatment, the patient will probably die or sustain permanent brain damage. Ara-A is ineffective against skin lesions.

Acycloguanosine, or acyclovir, does not cause unacceptable side effects when injected or applied to the skin. It may be one of the most promising agents yet discovered for treating the commonest forms of herpes, and it was licensed for use as an ointment in March 1982, and approval for intravenous administration is pending. Acyclovir is activated (by having a phosphate molecule attached to it) by the viral enzyme thymidine kinase. The same enzyme from normal cells is relatively inactive. Thus the activated form of the drug accumulates only in viral-infected cells, where it stops the synthesis of viral

DNA by an unknown mechanism. A second experimental drug, bromovinyldeoxyuridine, behaves similarly.

Two papers describing acyclovir treatment in immunosuppressed patients appeared in *The Lancet* for June 27, 1981, and the *New England Journal of Medicine* for July 9, 1981, respectively. Both described carefully designed clinical trials of acyclovir that were placebo-controlled and double-blind. In placebo-controlled trials, a group of patients is carefully matched to a second group for age, sex, and type of illness (among other things), and is treated exactly as the second group except that they are administered a harmless substance with no pharmacological effect instead of the drug under investigation. In a double-blind study, the investigator administering the drug or placebo does not know which is which; nor does the person who examines the patients for effects of the treatment. The patients are randomly assigned numbers, and only a third party, not otherwise involved in the trial, knows which is which. The results are tabulated according to the patients' numbers. Then, and only then, is the code broken that tells which patient received the drug under study and which received placebo. Such studies are expensive and time-consuming, but clinical trials carried out in any other way are generally useless.*

* The first clinical trial may have been that performed by the prophet Daniel, along with Shadrach, Meshach, and Abednego, during the Babylonian captivity. The four, not wanting to eat the meat and wine of King Nebuchadnezzar, suggested that they be allowed to consume a vegetarian diet for ten days, "Then let our countenances be looked upon before thee, and the countenance of the children that eat of the portion of the king's meat. . . ." At the end of ten days, the countenances of Daniel and his companions "appeared fairer and fatter in flesh than all the children which did eat the portion of the king's meat" (Daniel 1: 12–15). Daniel's study was, however, neither placebo-controlled nor double-blind.

Both these careful studies (and a more recent one described in the June 3, 1982, issue of the *New England Journal of Medicine*, where the subjects were otherwise healthy people with genital herpes) concluded that acyclovir was an effective agent for preventing and treating herpes infections, although there is still no drug known that will cure a latent herpes infection (that is, completely destroy the virus in the body), and a half-ounce of acyclovir ointment costs from $16 to $20. Trials indicate that intravenously administered acyclovir is even more effective than application as an ointment and this makes possible treatment of lesions in the urethra or on the cervix. Of course, acyclovir-resistant herpes virus was soon isolated from organ transplant patients treated with the drug.[12] But this story may have a happy ending. The acyclovir-resistant mutant HSV may cause much milder disease than the drug-susceptible virus and may, in fact, function as a live inactivated (attenuated) HSV vaccine.

Similarly, 2-deoxyglucose appears to "cure" genital herpes. It may, however, be toxic to the liver or heart. But all these, as well as many other drugs, are experimental and, with the exception of acyclovir, need much more investigation before they can be licensed for widespread use.

The protein interferon is naturally made in the body in response to viral infections. Although it is currently extremely expensive, it is becoming available as a result of genetic engineering in which the human gene for one type of interferon is transferred to a bacterium that then produces the protein in large quantities at low cost. Initial studies with interferon in the treatment of herpes looked promising, but subsequent investigations have not supported the original optimism. Other immune stimulants (Levamisol and Isoprinosine) are ineffectual and also dangerous.

Some viral diseases—smallpox, for example—have responded well to the development of a vaccine that immunizes a person against infection by the virus. This approach has naturally been considered for herpes and is still being pursued.

The problem is that even fragments of herpes virus are capable of causing tumors when injected into certain animals, and this fact casts a pall over efforts to develop a herpes vaccine. The same argument applies to killing the virus with various combinations of dye and light (usually ultraviolet). Light absorption may fragment the DNA of the virus so that it is no longer capable of producing herpes skin infection, but the fragmented virus may have even more dangerous properties. Once the genetics of this complex virus (which contains at least fifty-five genes compared with seven or eight for influenza viruses) is better understood, recombinant DNA technology may make it possible to prepare a live vaccine that is free of the tumor-producing genes.

A vaccine made of either isolated or synthetic viral coat protein(s) may soon be available, the subunit vaccine, but the central question of efficacy in humans remains unanswered. Merck, Sharpe and Dohme is currently carrying out human studies on their subunit vaccine, and other firms in the United States and Europe are similarly engaged. The risk of inducing malignancy with such a preparation is small.

Meanwhile, the suffering associated with genital herpes infections goes on, as interviews make clear:[13] "My first attack was so agonizing that I had to take two weeks sick leave . . . and handfuls of pain killers." "Herpes has cost me thousands of dollars, the loss of two wives (and children). . . . It has effectively destroyed my life. I no longer even bother with relationships at all." "I feel loathsome, worthless and untouchable as a sexual partner." "We think it's time some organization takes responsibility to do something about it."

There is such an organization, with some 30,000 members. It's called the Herpes Resource Center (formerly H E L P). For an $8.00 annual fee, a herpes sufferer may join and receive a quarterly journal on every aspect of herpes infection and answers to questions sent in by subscribers. Local chapters have meetings for their members. The Herpes Resource Center is run by the American Social Health Asso-

O Hateful Error, Melancholy's Child

"Life can be happy."

The interviewer persisted, "Is life happy?"

"You have to make it happy, don't you?" the boy replied.

"Are you happy?"

Eddie looked thoughtful for a moment. "There's nothing to make me sad."

Eddie Freeman, of Stevenage, in Hertsfordshire, England, was thirteen years old when this interview with NBC's George Montgomery took place in 1972. Eddie was born without arms or legs. He was going to an ordinary school in his wheelchair and drawing well with the two fingers attached to the short stump that serves as his right arm. In Eddie's view, it was much worse for people severely disabled in an accident since they knew what it was like to be normal. Although Eddie seemed devoid of self-pity, he would, if pressed, admit that he wished he could play games.

Carl Davies of London wanted to be a painter when first interviewed; although he has no arms, he has two fingers on a stump like Eddie Freeman. More recently, Carl has decided he would rather be a farmer. Carl rides horseback, swims, and bicycles—signaling a turn with the appropriate leg.

Philippa Bradborn wants to train horses. She likewise has no arms. She leads her horse by hooking one foot in its bridle, then hopping on the other foot until she has brought the animal alongside the stool she uses to climb into the saddle. Philippa was abandoned by her parents shortly after her birth and left to be raised by her grandparents. She said of her life in 1972 that there are "Not too many problems, really."

What these English children have in common, besides indomitable courage, is that their mothers took a mild sedative called Distaval between the fifth and the eighth week of their pregnancy. The drug was also called Softenon, Neurosedyn, Asmaval, Tensival, Valgraine, Kevadon, Contergan, Sedalis, and forty-two other trade names. Dr. Wilhelm Kunz, who first synthesized the sedative, had been a sergeant in the German Army during World War II. Like many veterans after the war, he continued his education and became a pharmacist, then went to work for the small firm of Chemie Grünenthal in the town of Stolberg-im-Rhein, some ten kilometers (six miles) east of Aachen.

After Kunz had made and purified the compound, he determined its chemical properties. As he presumably wrote in his notebook (none of the laboratory notebooks recording Chemie Grünenthal's work on this substance has ever been found), it was a white crystalline powder, odorless and tasteless, that melted at between 269° and 271°C. It was insoluble in both ether and benzene and only slightly soluble in water, ethyl or methyl alcohol, or glacial acetic acid. Chemically, it was called N-(2,6-dioxo-3 piperidyl) pthalimide. The general public knows this substance better as thalidomide.

Chemie Grünenthal's enthusiastic and totally unscrupulous marketing of thalidomide led to the birth of more than

8,000 severely deformed children in 46 countries around the world, and to the stillbirths, spontaneous abortions, or early postnatal deaths of uncounted others. The thalidomide story is an instructive saga of corporate deceit, treachery, and greed that is sickening to contemplate even more than twenty years later.

On Tuesday, October 1, 1957, thalidomide went on sale to the German public over the counter, rather than by prescription, and accompanied by a massive advertising campaign describing Contergan (as thalidomide was called in Germany) as "astonishingly safe," "fully harmless," and "non-toxic." This was palpable nonsense. Chemie Grünenthal was lying—and they knew it. At the Grünenthal symposium at Stolberg-im-Rhein in mid-December 1955, nearly two years before marketing began, a number of physicians had reported potentially serious side effects of the drug.

Nevertheless, thalidomide was exported to 11 European, 7 African, 17 Asian, and 11 North and South American countries, accompanied by 50 advertisements in major medical journals, 200,000 letters sent to physicians, and 50,000 circulars sent to pharmacists. Each of these, as well as the instruction leaflet accompanying each bottle, referred to the drug as "completely safe."[1] Pharmacologists and some physicians around the world knew that there was no such thing as an effective drug that was "completely safe," but for the most part, the medical profession uncritically embraced this apparent miracle with enthusiasm. Sales of thalidomide soared beyond Chemie Grünenthal's wildest dreams.

Some physicians scattered thalidomide tablets among their patients in double handfuls and kept no records of how much and to whom. But more thoughtful and observant doctors were beginning to have second thoughts. A year after thalidomide's release, German physicians began writing to Stolberg-im-Rhein reporting dizziness and disturbance of balance in some patients. Later, they frequently reported the more serious side effect of peripheral neuritis. To all these letters and telephone calls the medical staff at Chemie Grünenthal had a standard answer: "This is the first time such side effects have been reported to us."

By autumn 1958, reports of peripheral neuritis were clattering down on Chemie Grünenthal like hailstones. Peripheral neuritis is a grave ailment. Prickling begins in the hands and feet, followed by numbness and cold, severe cramps, weakness, and loss of coordination since the victim can no longer feel where his or her feet are. Even after Grünenthal grudgingly admitted that peripheral neuritis was a demonstrable side effect of thalidomide, they claimed that, in the occasional patient who suffered from the ailment, the condition cleared as soon as the medication was stopped. This was yet another lie. Occasionally, the neuritis slowly disappeared over several years after treatment with thalidomide was stopped; but more often the victims were permanently disabled. Later, a young tennis coach in England committed suicide after thalidomide-induced neuritis robbed him of his livelihood.

The door to the thalidomide chamber of horrors now stood ajar. It would soon swing fully open to reveal the ghastly results of corporate indifference, ineptitude, and greed.

In 1956, Chemie Grünenthal had tried to sell an American license for thalidomide to Smith, Kline & French (SKF). The SKF research laboratory in Philadelphia carefully tested the drug, concluded that it had no useful properties, and turned it down. Unfortunately, less competent companies were seduced by the siren song of the Stolberg-im-Rhein maidens and bought licenses to distribute thalidomide.

One such company was Distillers Co. Ltd. Distillers has a near monopoly on the worldwide distribution of British Scotch, gin, and other liquors, and is one of England's largest and richest companies. After World War II, the British government offered Distillers a penicillin plant at a price they couldn't refuse, and Distillers formed Distillers Company (Biochemicals) Limited—DCBL—as the penicillin-producing branch of the company. Penicillin production was never very profitable. By the mid-1950s, Distillers wanted to expand into more lucrative lines like the marketing of synthetic drugs. The simplest procedure was to buy a license for a drug already developed by a foreign company. Thus Distillers joined Chemie Grünenthal and the blind began leading the blind.

Grünenthal, an offshoot of a soap and cosmetics firm, was itself a "Johann-come-lately" to the highly sophisticated world of drug synthesis. Chemie Grünenthal, like DCBL, was formed to cash in on the vast postwar market for antimicrobial drugs (antibiotics) produced by various molds. Like DCBL, Chemie Grünenthal decided to enter the drug synthesis business in the mid-1950s, which they did by hiring a half dozen scientists and technicians and putting them to work. Thalidomide was one of the first products of this new effort. It showed some activity as a sedative and appeared to be only very slightly toxic, since even very high doses did not kill rats. No effort was ever made by Grünenthal to determine how thalidomide exerted its effects or how it was metabolized and excreted; no tests on pregnant animals were ever performed.

The so-called clinical trials of thalidomide were a cruel farce. The drug was given to physicians who were, for the most part, receiving retainers from Chemie Grünenthal. They were asked to try it on their patients and let Grünenthal know their impressions. Most of these physicians gave the experimental drug to a few patients for periods ranging from a couple of days to a couple of weeks. For the most part, in these very restricted circumstances, the drug seemed mildly effective and quite harmless, although some doctors reported side effects that would have caused a more principled firm to make a careful investigation before rushing to market.

Not so Chemie Grünenthal. In October 1957, Contergan went on the market over the counter as a mild sedative and tranquilizer. Grünenthal was responsible for producing all the thalidomide sold in the world. Its licensees were supplied with the drug made in Stolberg, out of which they could make tablets and syrups, or combine thalidomide with other drugs as they saw fit.

Distillers Biochemical representatives visiting Chemie Grünenthal were easily persuaded that thalidomide was a fabulous product. In England at that time, about a million people took some sort of pill each night to help them sleep; every eighth prescription written under the National Health Plan was for a sedative.[2] Thalidomide, marketed in England through DCBL as Distaval, became available on April 14, 1958. Three years later, DCBL sent British doctors a pamphlet alleging that Distaval could be given to pregnant women without adverse effect on either mother or child. That there was not a shred of evidence to support this claim seemed to bother DCBL as little as it had bothered Chemie Grünenthal, which had originated the statement without having done any investigations to determine whether or not it was true.

By mid-1960, DCBL had reports on five patients who had developed peripheral polyneuritis after prolonged use of Distaval. The New Year's Eve issue of the *British Medical Journal* carried a letter by Dr. A. Leslie Florence of Turriff, Aberdeenshire, who reported four cases of peripheral polyneuritis following Distaval treatment. This was the first published account of the serious side effect. Although it had been observed in Germany for several years, the information was not made public, at least in part because of determined efforts by Chemie Grünenthal to suppress it.

By July 1961, Distillers Biochemical knew of over a hundred cases of peripheral neuritis and of one suicide by an overdose of Distaval. By October, DCBL was aware of a total of 130 cases of peripheral neuritis, yet in the following month's *British Medical Journal* a DCBL advertisement claimed: "There is no case on record in which even a gross overdosage with Distaval has had harmful results. . . . Depend on the safety of Distaval."

The American market still shimmered like a vast sea of gold before the eyes of Chemie Grünenthal's managers. After

Smith, Kline & French turned them down, they tried Lederle, and were turned down again. Then in the autumn of 1958, Richardson-Merrell signed agreements with Chemie Grünenthal to market thalidomide in the United States.

Richardson-Merrell, although one of the country's largest drug companies, was not in the first rank of American pharmaceutical firms. It was, however, on an ethical par with DCBL and Grünenthal. On February 11, 1959, Richardson-Merrell began distributing Kevadon (its name for thalidomide) to private physicians for experimental use on their patients. Three months later it expanded the clinical trials to include pregnant women, although it had precisely as much information on thalidomide effects during pregnancy as had DCBL and Chemie Grünenthal—namely, none.

After the clinical trials were under way, Richardson-Merrell began thalidomide experiments on laboratory animals. Although the company had done studies on pregnant animals with its previous "wonder drug"—called Mer 29—they did none on Kevadon. Richardson-Merrell scientists did learn that thalidomide syrup was quickly lethal to rats and dogs. DCBL had known this too, but that hadn't stopped Grünenthal from marketing the syrup in Germany as a sedative for babies. And, despite the test results, Richardson-Merrell went on with large-scale clinical trials preparatory to applying to the FDA for permission to market the drug. More than 2.5 million thalidomide tablets were given to nearly 1,300 physicians, who, in turn, passed them on to some 20,000 patients. Salesmen were told not to offer the physicians the placebos (fake pills) that were an essential part of a scientifically valid clinical trial unless the physicians specifically asked for them; and the salesmen did not distribute the consent forms that the American Medical Association had devised, and that were supposed to be signed by a patient to whom an experimental drug was given.

Thalidomide Day in the United States was set for March 6, 1961, at which time the drug would be launched at an unsuspecting public on a tidal wave of publicity. The application to the FDA arrived at the agency on September 12, 1960, and was routed to a newly arrived medical officer for evaluation. Frances Kelsey, M.D., Ph.D., then forty-six, was both a physician and a pharmacologist. Canadian-born, she and her husband, also a pharmacologist, had just joined the FDA staff after moving to Washington from Vermillion, South Dakota.

Frances Kelsey spent a month examining the Kevadon application in great detail. She didn't like what she saw. Neither animal nor clinical studies were reported in sufficient detail to allow any conclusions to be drawn, and an insufficient number of human cases had been studied. In a drug absorption study in which a statistically significant number of rats had been treated, the data did not, in Dr. Kelsey's opinion, support the conclusion Richardson-Merrell had drawn. The company's data on chronic toxicity, drug stability, and side effects were all inadequate. (Late in 1960, an internal FDA document written by Frances Kelsey's husband characterized one section of Richardson-Merrell's application as an "interesting collection of meaningless, pseudoscientific jargon . . ." and commented in another section that "the data are completely meaningless as presented.")[8]

Richardson-Merrell kept pressuring the FDA to release Kevadon, and Dr. Frances Kelsey kept demanding more convincing data on the drug's safety. Then, in late February 1961, Richardson-Merrell's hopes of marketing Kevadon in the United States began to crumble when Frances Kelsey saw Dr. Florence's letter in the *British Medical Journal* on thalidomide and peripheral neuritis. She suspected, quite correctly, that Richardson-Merrell had known about the problem all along. In a telephone conversation with the company's medical contact man with the FDA, she gave him a chance to volunteer the information she was certain he had by asking leading questions. He said nothing about polyneuritis.

To meet Dr. Kelsey's objections, two of the Richardson-

Merrell medical staff flew to Stolberg-im-Rhein for a consultation. They then reported to Frances Kelsey that Chemie Grünenthal knew of only thirty-four cases of peripheral neuritis in Germany and that all of these had cleared up immediately when thalidomide treatment was stopped. Dr. Kelsey was skeptical, as well she might have been. By that time Grünenthal actually knew of 400 cases of peripheral neuritis and was aware that the side effect was often irreversible. Dr. Kelsey had also made the very important point to Richardson-Merrell that since thalidomide was only another entry in an already crowded field of reasonably safe and effective sedatives, the presence of a serious side effect associated with its use would be entirely unacceptable.

By November 1961, more than a year after the original submission of their application on Kevadon, Richardson-Merrell still had not convinced Dr. Frances Kelsey that the drug could be safely marketed. Then, on Saturday, November 18, 1961, at a pediatrics meeting in Düsseldorf, two German pediatricians, Drs. Kosenow and Pfeiffer, described thirty-four infants with limb defects that they had seen in the past two years at the Children's Hospital, Münster. Some of the assembled physicians remembered that, two months earlier, Dr. H. R. Weidemann had reported on thirteen similar cases seen in just ten months, and a still earlier case had been reported by Dr. A. Weidenbach in November 1959 in which a child was born without arms or legs—but the cause of all these cases had remained a mystery.

At this point, Prof. Dr. Widukind Lenz, head of the Children's Clinic of Hamburg University, stood up after Kosenow and Pfeiffer's paper to report on fourteen children born with severe deformities whose mothers had taken "a certain substance" during pregnancy. Later he told his close associates at the meeting that the substance was thalidomide.

On December 16, 1961, the weekly British medical journal *The Lancet* carried a letter from a Sydney, Australia, obstetrician, Dr. William McBride, reporting severely deformed children born to nearly 20 percent of mothers who had taken thalidomide during pregnancy. Ironically, McBride had written a paper for *The Lancet* in mid-June pointing out the high incidence of severe and multiple birth defects in a large proportion of the offspring of mothers taking thalidomide, but the editors had deemed it insufficiently convincing to publish.

Chemie Grünenthal withdrew thalidomide from the German market on Monday, November 27, 1961, after having sold the drug for more than four years. Distillers Biochemical followed less than a week later, and Richardson-Merrell's application to market the drug in the United States promptly sank out of sight.

Although thalidomide was withdrawn in Germany and Great Britain, it would be months before the last children deformed by the drug were born. In the United States, where it had never been marketed, there were at least sixteen thalidomide babies born subsequent to the Richardson-Merrell clinical trials. At that time abortion was illegal in all fifty states, so a woman knowing that she might bear a severely deformed child had no legal recourse but to wait and see. Sherry Finkbine, a Phoenix television personality, made a much-publicized trip to Sweden to get an abortion, but for most American women who knew that they had taken thalidomide and were now informed of its grisly potential through their newspapers, pregnancy was transformed from a period of joyful expectation to one of terror and uncertainty.

Elsewhere things were even worse. The drug was promptly removed from the market in Sweden, but since the Swedish authorities did not warn women against thalidomide pills already released, the tragic result was the birth of at least five babies needlessly crippled. In Japan, the situation was appalling. The drug continued to be sold over the counter for more than a year; the inevitable result was the birth of several hundred severely deformed children to Japanese mothers. In Italy, thalidomide was on the market ten months after its withdrawal from the German and British markets, and it took three months for the governments of Argentina and Canada to remove the drug from circulation. The Argentinian victims were supplied with the drug by a Swedish company that callously continued to sell the compound in Argentina for months after it had been withdrawn in Sweden. The fate of thalidomide in several dozen other countries is unknown. It is likely that in most of them the drug remained on the market until the supply was exhausted and no more could be obtained.

The next chapter in the thalidomide story—the attempt by the victims to get reparations from the manufacturers to relieve them of some of the crushing financial burdens of caring for severely disabled children—is as sordid a story of corporate and governmental indifference as was that of the drug's initial promotion and distribution.

Only in Germany did the government take on the burden of acting on behalf of the parents of thalidomide children to force adequate compensation from Chemie Grünenthal for its criminal negligence. Because Chemie Grünenthal refused to give them up voluntarily, important documents had to be seized in police raids. Even then, essential evidence was apparently destroyed by the company to prevent its use in court.

On September 2, 1965, the German federal prosecutor charged nine Grünenthal executives with intent to commit bodily harm and involuntary manslaughter. That was only the preliminary indictment. The complete indictment took two more years to complete and spanned nearly 1,000 pages. It would be a trial on the same scale, and with the same emotional impact, as Nuremberg, and for much the same sort of behavior.

The trial lasted two years and seven months before Grünenthal agreed to compensate the victims at a modest level rather than continue the protracted fight in court. The victims (some 5,000 in all) got $31 million from Grünenthal and nearly the same amount from the German government. They also had the advantage of living in a society in which superb medical care has been freely available for nearly a century. Although the settlement was modest, it was at least timely. For many of the thalidomide victims elsewhere, the judicial system failed miserably. In presumably enlightened Sweden it was eight years after the drug had been withdrawn before Swedish victims were modestly compensated.

In the United Kingdom, as almost everywhere else except Germany and Sweden, the parents of thalidomide children were left to their own devices. The English laws on contempt of court effectively deprived the parents of their most effective weapon against Distillers when it denied them newspaper or television coverage of their struggle; the legal battle against Distillers took ten years before the company agreed to compensate the victims of its own ineptitude and avarice.

In the United States, things went better for the thalidomide victims, thanks to three peculiarities in the American legal system. The first of these is the strict liability laws; the second is the ability (increasingly abused) of American lawyers to take cases on a contingency fee basis—that is, if they lose the case they get nothing, whereas if they win they get a substantial portion (up to one half) of the settlement. The third factor is a thoroughly free press that cannot be prevented, as it was in Britain, from discussing cases being tried in court.

Twenty years after the disaster, the thalidomide victims and their parents (victims as well) continue to bear a ghastly burden that no financial compensation, no matter how generous, can ever completely allay. The three English children mentioned in the beginning of this chapter were all born without arms. This meant that their mothers took thalidomide between the twenty-fifth and thirtieth day of pregnancy. Other children affected during this period had severely shortened arms, fused or supernumerary fingers, or hands attached to their arms at unusual angles.

Children whose mothers took thalidomide between the twentieth and twenty-fourth day of pregnancy had ear and eye defects and paralysis of their facial and cranial nerves that left them deformed and, in some cases, deaf and blind as well. Other children were born with severe brain damage.

Children with lower limb defects resulted when their mothers took the drug from the thirty-first to the thirty-fourth day of pregnancy. The defects ranged from shortening of the bones and supernumerary toes to dislocated hips, deformed pelvis, club feet, and total absence of one or both legs. One unfortunate woman took a single 200 milligram tablet of thalidomide during this period and later had a child with severely shortened arms and legs.

Other children were born with visceral defects that were corrected surgically, but a still greater number with such defects were either born dead or died within a few days of birth. Children of mothers who took thalidomide over a prolonged period during pregnancy were born with nearly all possible defects. Some of them survive today.

Peggy McCarrick was born while her mother was still in a Los Angeles high school. Peggy's short right leg ended in a flipper, her hip joints were malformed, and she had bladder and anal abnormalities. After repeated operations, she now gets around well on an artificial leg and is financially reasonably well off because of the reparations she received from Richardson-Merrell.

Terry Wiles, the illegitimate English son of a white mother and a black father, has neither arms nor legs. Two flippers extend from his lower body; one has three digits, the other four. He has no pelvic bones, and at birth one eye hung halfway down his cheek and had to be removed. Abandoned, he spent six years in a hospital for handicapped children. Today, he is just over 2 feet tall. Adopted by a loving couple, Terry writes short stories with his toes on a special electric typewriter at twenty-seven words a minute, reads extensively, plays the electric organ, makes and flies model aircraft, and holds his own at the business college he attends. His short-hand speed is fifty words a minute.

These are inspiring testimonies to human courage and endurance. But others of the thalidomide children are blind, deaf, dumb, severely paralyzed, and hopelessly retarded. Some of them still live with their parents, who face the daily tasks of changing diapers on a twenty-two-year-old, or lifting a 125-pound child from a wheelchair into a taxi so that the child can go to school. Some of the parents have institution-alized children whom they cannot bear to see, and all the mothers must face the realization that if they had not taken that one, or two, or three little white pills to help them sleep some twenty years ago they might still be living normal lives.

This crushing burden of guilt has twisted the lives of wives and husbands as surely as the bodies of their children have grown awry. Compensation has been paid to the chil-dren, not their parents, so that some of the children own— or soon will own—the homes in which they live. They can, if they choose, turn their parents out of doors, and some of them, in their anger and pain, have threatened to do just that.

We've seen some of the havoc wrought by thalidomide. Now we need to examine the simple statement: thalidomide causes limb reduction deformities (blocked limb development). Does this mean that all such defects were caused by thalidomide? Certainly not. Limb reductions occurred long before thalido-mide and they continue to occur. Does the statement mean that thalidomide always causes reduction deformities in the offspring of women who have take it during the critical period of pregnancy? The answer is again no. Some women (a small proportion) apparently took thalidomide without ill effects on the child they were carrying. Teratogens (compounds capable of causing birth defects) almost never cause 100 per-cent incidence of abnormalities in the animals (human or otherwise) to which they are administered. Hence the concept of multifactorialness—that a birth defect results from exposure to a sufficient dose of teratogen at a critical period of intrauterine development *plus* a susceptibility factor or factors that cause one mother-fetus pair to respond by producing a birth defect where another pair would not. This concept, which applies to cancer causality as well, makes the study and prevention of birth defects extraordinarily complicated.

Of course, birth defects neither began nor ended with thalidomide. Prehistoric cave paintings depict malformed children. A figurine dating from about 6500 b.c. shows a figure with two heads on one body. To the teratologist—a student of birth defects—this is a not uncommon malformation; to the superstitious, it was a twin goddess. Drawings of similar figures abound. A huge example in New South Wales, Australia, shows a double-headed male figure with four left and six right fingers.[4] A book printed in 1642 shows a child with a "thalidomide-like" deformity. The left arm is missing, the right has a hand with three fingers attached by a short stump to the shoulder. An adult male pictured in the same volume has a shortened left arm terminating in a clubbed hand with only two fingers, and severely deformed and shortened legs. Dürer woodcuts (1512) and a painting by Goya, among many other artistic representations, show children with malformations.

At present, approximately ten children of every hundred are born with some congenital malformation. These range from trivial to devastating. The first abdominal surgery I ever witnessed was performed on a sixteen-year-old girl with a mysterious abdominal mass that everyone feared would be malignant. It was, in fact, a second uterus and the problem was readily solved. A sixty-two-year-old Los Alamos, New Mexico, woman with a urethral stone was recently found on examination to have an extra ureter. This had complicated the problem of finding the stone but had not caused any other problems for six decades. Many "malformations"—birthmarks normally covered by clothing, for example—are even more trivial. The interesting questions are what causes birth defects, particularly the serious ones, and how can they be prevented?

The view is widespread, even in the medical profession, that birth defects have only two causes: drugs and chemicals. This is not true.

There is no particular agreement among teratologists about the proportion of causes of various birth defects, but the consensus is not far from that offered by Dr. F. Clarke Fraser of McGill University, Montreal.[5] In his view, about one birth defect in twenty is caused by a mutation (other estimates are as much as seven times higher), while two in twenty result from a microscopically visible chromosomal abnormality (unlike mutations, in which the damage to the DNA of the gene is submicroscopic). Dr. Fraser estimates that approximately four of every twenty birth defects result from the multifactorial combination of a particular insult to the developing fetus (exposure to a toxic chemical, for example) and a genetic susceptibility to that insult. If either the insult or the susceptibility is lacking, no birth defect results. Professor Fraser has given estimates for the causes of about 40 percent of all birth defects. Teratologists may argue about the distribution of causes—one view is that radiation, viruses, drugs, and chemicals combined account for no more than 10 percent of all birth defects[6]—but there is general agreement that we have no idea what causes a substantial proportion of them.

Birth defects are far more common than is generally realized, because nature, the great abortionist, rejects most of them. At least one half of all human pregnancies terminate in spontaneous abortion, and over 70 percent of the aborted fetuses are seriously malformed. It is clear that the incidence of severe birth defects is very high indeed. When these birth defects are incompatible with continued intrauterine development, the damaged fetuses are spontaneously aborted. The defects that are compatible with life in the protected environment of the womb, but not compatible with life outside it, are responsible for 20 percent of the infant mortality in the United States since the child dies at, or shortly after, birth.

It is clear that the first line of defense against the birth of damaged children is spontaneous abortion. Where rates of spontaneous abortion are high, live births of deformed children are low, and vice versa. Were it not for this natural selection, the incidence of serious birth defects in live-born children would be many times higher than it is. Development of a drug that would enhance the spontaneous abortion of defective fetuses would be one approach to reducing birth defects and postnatal infant mortality.

If "drugs and chemicals" were a major contributor to the incidence of birth defects, we might expect to see a steady increase in the incidence of birth defects as more and more women are exposed to both.[7] As part of their Birth Defects Monitoring Program, experts at the CDC have collected data for nearly one third of the children born in the United States each year on the incidence of 161 categories of birth defects. These data are analyzed quarterly to determine trends that would suggest either the introduction of a powerful new teratogen or of a means for preventing a class of malformations.

In a recent report, the CDC statisticians compared the incidence, between 1970 and 1977, of sixteen birth defects that occurred in sufficient numbers to form a reliable basis for analysis, could be readily diagnosed, and involved a variety of organ systems. Their overall conclusion was that "In the period covered in this report the incidence of the majority of birth defects neither substantially decreased nor increased."[8]

Christopher Norwood, in her book *At Highest Risk*, writes of the increasing rate of spontaneous abortion as yet another index, with the "increasing" incidence of birth defects, of mounting exposure of pregnant women to drugs and chemicals.[9] The rate of spontaneous abortion, however, for a group of over 2,000 University of Minnesota women studied between 1935 and 1944 was nearly identical with that of an age-matched group of 1,375 women from the university studied a generation later (1961 to 1970).[10] Neither the incidence of birth defects nor spontaneous abortion seem to have increased in recent years.

In a recent report from Japan that also casts doubt on the relationship between occupational exposure to chemicals and birth defects, the lowest proportion of malformed embryos was found in women who were industrial workers; the highest proportion was found in clerical workers.[11]

Many compounds that are carcinogens (cancer-producing) are also capable of producing birth defects, and there is talk of a "cancer epidemic" sweeping the United States, most often connected with the irresponsible disposal of carcinogenic chemical wastes.[12] Love Canal is the most frequently cited example of a situation in which large numbers of innocent people whose homes were built over a buried industrial dump were exposed to very dangerous chemical wastes, resulting in an outbreak of cancer and birth defects.

That disposal of chemical wastes has been, and is, frequently irresponsible is unquestioned. That this may at some time have an influence on the rates of cancer incidence is entirely possible. At the moment, however, there is little evidence for a "cancer epidemic" in the United States other than that caused by cigarette smoking (the estimated source of about one-third of all cancer).[13] The incidence of most types of cancer (excluding lung), like that of most birth defects, fluctuates slightly but shows little change in the overall rates over the past three or four decades.[14] If there is any long-term trend in the incidence of both birth defects and cancer in the United States, it is probably downward.

According to the New York State Department of Health, the cancer rate has not increased in Love Canal residents.[15] There is also no evidence yet of an increase in the incidence of birth defects in the children of parents living near Love

Canal. That children with birth defects have been born to mothers in the Love Canal area is unequivocal, but, as we have seen, the chance of having a child with a serious birth defect that will markedly handicap the child if it cannot be corrected is at least one in fifty. With such a high background, data on a very large number of births must be collected before it can be said with any conviction that the incidence of birth defects has either increased or decreased in a statistically significant way.

For example, if a scientist suspects that a particular agent doubles the frequency of a birth defect that appears in 1 of every 1,000 births, he or she would have to study the offspring of at least 23,000 women exposed to the agent to obtain convincing evidence of cause and effect. No such study has been, or probably ever will be, carried out. It would take years and cost millions of dollars.

In the case of thalidomide, obtaining evidence of cause and effect was simpler since the defects commonly observed were those that most pediatricians and obstetricians had never seen before in a lifetime of practice. A doubling in the incidence of common defects like club foot, cleft palate, and Down syndrome would be much more difficult to detect. Fortunately, it's a hallmark of teratogens that a given compound produces a specific defect or group of defects, rather than simply increasing the number of a broad spectrum of defects. For example, tetracyclines given during pregnancy may produce mottled teeth in the offspring; streptomycin given during pregnancy may cause deafness. Neither agent results in any other kind of malformation.

The collection of small amounts of birth defect data can lead to completely misleading results. The distribution of severe birth defects seen at a rambling late Victorian-style hospital in an inner suburb of Sydney, Australia, in early 1961 is one such example. The hospital is known locally as Crown Street, but its official name is the Woman's Hospital, Sydney. Crown Street handles some 4,000 deliveries a year, and at the beginning of 1961, Dr. John Newlinds, the medical superintendent, was a very worried man. Crown Street's rate of congenital malformations was about three times the national average and close to five times that observed in Australia's second largest woman's hospital in Melbourne.

Dr. Newlinds bought a large map of Sydney and began sticking pins in it to locate the home of each malformed child. He soon had a dense cluster of pins in an area south of Sydney known as Lucas Heights. The interesting thing about Lucas Heights was that a nuclear power reactor was located there, and Dr. Newlinds wondered if radiation was connected with the severe birth defects. But six months later he photographed the map, took out the pins, and put the map away.

By then Dr. Newlinds had the answer, or part of it. The density of pins represented the number of women in the area who had gone to Crown Street to have their babies. "The areas with a lot of pins were areas where the doctors liked us and sent their patients to us. It was as simple as that."[16] It was only later that it became apparent that the high malformation rate at Crown Street was due to the use of thalidomide there as a result of Distillers' determination to distribute the drug in what is one of the largest women's hospitals in the southern hemisphere. Fortunately, Dr. Newlinds had waited until he had more data before leading a mob to shut down the Lucas Heights reactor. Someone less well trained might not have been so patient. In the area of birth defects, as in so many others, inadequate data may be worse than no data at all.

The Love Canal disaster has much in common with the Crown Street experience, and is in many ways analogous to the incident at Three Mile Island. In each case there was corporate blundering, technological catastrophe, and a crushing burden of fear and foreboding laid upon innocent bystanders. Anyone who has seen television interviews with the homeowners at Love Canal is painfully aware that many of them are terrified and miserable. Yet at Love Canal, as at Three Mile Island, the principal damage suffered by the area's residents may be the result of a long period of terror and uncertainty, for the creation and promulgation of which the news media bear a considerable responsibility.*

The time lag between exposure to a carcinogen and the appearance of human cancer is often measured in decades. So an increased incidence of cancer in the residents of Love Canal may not be evident until the end of this century. Increases in birth defects, on the other hand, can be detected within a few years. No such increases have yet appeared in the Love Canal residents, although their emotional suffering has been painful almost beyond endurance.

On the important question of the relationship between industrial chemicals and human health, the words of Joshua Lederberg—geneticist, Nobel Laureate, and president of Rockefeller University—in a speech to the United Nations Association early in 1981, are worth pondering. "With all of the enormous expansion both in quality and quantity—that is, in the variety and total material—of the chemical industry, I believe today that we're in a far healthier position than we were thirty years ago. . . . With respect to a wide variety of substances, I am quite confident that the average exposure to many of these chemicals is down by a factor of 100 or 1,000 compared to what it was in the early 1950s, just on account of the awareness that has been generated, the public

* Lewis Thomas, M.D., chaired a panel of five distinguished physicians appointed by the governor of New York to assess the (more or less) scientific studies on Love Canal. In his letter of transmittal of the panel's report to Governor Carey, Dr. Thomas wrote that "the Panel has concluded that there has been no demonstration of acute health effects linked to exposure to hazardous wastes at the Love Canal site." The panel did not rule out possible long-term effects. (A copy of the letter and of the panel's report were kindly provided by Dr. Thomas.)

sensitivities about these matters. . . . This is an enormous advance over what was the case thirty years ago."

Whatever the cause, birth defects are common, and the knowledge that their unborn child may be seriously defective brings to parents the most agonizing questions they will ever be forced to answer.

Down syndrome (mongolism), for example, is caused by the appearance of an extra chromosome or part of a chromosome at position 21, and is readily detectable by amniocentesis, that is, the removal of a small amount of the amniotic fluid surrounding the fetus, which contains fetal cells. The probability of a twenty-five-year-old woman having a child with Down syndrome is 1 in 2,000 or less, but the risk increases several-fold for each decade thereafter; about 1 in every 40 offspring of a forty-five-year-old woman would have this chromosomal aberration. About 5,000 American children with Down syndrome are born each year. Fortunately, the incidence dropped steadily until the 1970s (as the proportion of births to women over thirty-five decreased);[17] about 70 percent of fetuses with Down syndrome are lost by spontaneous abortion. Although a report in the *American Journal of Epidemiology* for June 1982 ruled out environmental factors as a cause of Down syndrome, the authors expect the number of Down syndrome births to rise steadily throughout the 1980s as the large cohort of women born in the post–World War II baby boom have their last children.

Children with this defect are frequently good-natured and pleasant, but they are often so severely retarded that they require life-long institutional care at a cost that approaches $0.5 million. These children frequently die in their teens of respiratory and heart problems, or in their twenties of leukemia. If they survive those hazards, their lives are often cut short by the premature development of a progressive senile dementia resembling Alzheimer's disease. Many of the afflicted children are born with portions of their intestine pinched off;

they must be operated on immediately or they'll die. If, despite all these problems, the parents elect to care for their child at home, they face the subsequent problem of who will take care of it when they are dead or too old or sick to do so themselves.

Tay-Sachs disease represents an entirely different problem. Here the loss of a single enzyme (hexosamidase A) leads to accumulation of lipid deposits in the brain, causing its rapid degeneration. A Tay-Sachs child may be normal for the first six months of its life or even longer, but then quickly deteriorates both physically and mentally, becoming blind, helpless, and eventually dying as a vegetable, often before the age of five.

Fortunately for diagnostic purposes, the disease is confined to the descendants of eastern European Jews, which includes about 90 percent of American Jews. The chance of both parents in an American Jewish household having the genetic disorder is about 1 in 900, and the test for the disease is relatively simple. A person carrying the gene for Tay-Sachs disease has only half the blood level of hexosamidase A of a noncarrier. In one study of 10,000 people, both partners in only 11 couples had the Tay-Sachs gene. Five of those women became pregnant and all opted for amniocentesis; one Tay-Sachs fetus was detected and aborted. The other four couples, now free of the fear of having a child with this heartbreaking defect, had normal children.

The Tay-Sachs story is one of the modest triumphs in the battle to prevent the birth of seriously malformed children. Another success story is that associated with the greatly decreasing incidence of the congenital rubella (German measles) syndrome.

In 1941, following a rubella epidemic, the Australian opthalmologist N. W. Gregg described a sudden increase in the number of babies born with cataracts. Later it became clear that a pregnant woman who had rubella, particularly during the first trimester of pregnancy, risked having a child with cataracts, abnormally small head or eyes, mental retardation, blindness, deafness, heart disease, and a variety of other lesions of the bones and internal organs. About 20 percent of such afflicted children die within their first two years of life.

Fifty percent of women who have rubella during the first month of pregnancy will have children with rubella syndrome. If a woman is infected in the second month of pregnancy, the chance of having such a child drops to one in four, while infection in the next three months reduces the odds to one in ten or less.

This dreadful outcome can be simply prevented by effectively immunizing girls with rubella vaccine, preferably before they enter their child-bearing years. Such a vaccine became available in 1969. Before that, a woman who had rubella, especially during her first month of pregnancy, had the agonizing choice of whether or not to have an abortion, legal or otherwise. Fortunately, before 1969, most cases of German measles occurred in school-age children.

Now, however, at least 70 percent of rubella cases occur in people who are fifteen years or older, and the vaccination of adolescents and young adults is necessary to eliminate rubella syndrome. In January 1979, rubella vaccine grown in cultured human cells became available and the problems associated with the previous duck embryo cell vaccine (caused by traces of duck protein) became a thing of the past. The CDC Advisory Committee on Immunization Practices (ACIP) believes that the new vaccine is so safe it can even be given in pregnancy since, based on the limited experience thus far available, the vaccine virus does not appear in the fetus, as it frequently did with the older vaccines. Over a hundred women who had been vaccinated with the new vaccine from three months before to three months after conception went to term; none had children that exhibited any component of the rubella syndrome. Nevertheless, the ACIP recommends that the vaccine not be given to a woman known to be pregnant and that a woman receiving the vaccine avoid becoming pregnant until three months after her vaccination. Immunity following vaccination is, according to the ACIP, probably life-long.[18] Unfortunately, as of April 1982, twelve states (Hawaii, Idaho, Utah, Wyoming, Kansas, Louisiana, Kentucky, West Virginia, Virginia, Michigan, Pennsylvania, and New Hampshire) still have school immunization laws that are inadequate to protect young women from this disease.

The effect of rubella vaccination on the incidence of the disease has been striking. In 1978, there were over 18,000 cases, nearly 90 percent in people over fifteen. The following year, there were fewer than 12,000 cases; and in 1980, there were under 4,000 reported cases (much rubella goes unreported since it is often a very mild disease). In 1981, there was a further drop to some 3,000 cases. According to the *Morbidity and Mortality Weekly Report* of May 7, 1982, the ACIP hopes to eliminate indigenous measles in the United States by October 1982; Canada has a similar objective. The United States seems well on the way: by the third week of September 1982 only 1,230 cases of measles were reported, more than 50 percent fewer than for the same period in 1981.

The reductions of Tay-Sachs disease and rubella syndrome are milestones in preventing the birth of severely defective children. Yet the sickle cell screening program was a spectacular fiasco.

One American black in 600 has sickle cell anemia, a disease that ranges from trivial to severe. This uncertain outcome reduces the justification for abortion so that identifying fetuses with the disease is of dubious benefit. About one black in twelve has sickle cell trait—that is, he or she has one sickle cell gene and one normal gene. Carriers of sickle cell trait are generally healthy. The mass screening programs of the late 1960s did little to prevent and nothing to improve treatment of the disease. The principal result was to stigmatize carriers of sickle cell trait as "sick" because other people confused the trait with the disease. Carriers lost their jobs, were unable to obtain others, and were charged higher insurance premiums because of their supposed illness. The only accomplishment of the sickle cell screening program was unfairly to categorize and frighten some 2 million people.

An informed woman can find plenty of things to worry about. But two hazards, although much in the news, are probably not worth worrying over. One is diethylstilbesterol (DES), once commonly given to prevent miscarriage and now known to produce cervical or vaginal cancer in some of the adult daughters of women who took it during pregnancy. DES is the only compound yet known to produce transplacental carcinogenesis in humans; that is, it is capable of crossing the placental barrier and causing cancer in some of the offspring decades later. Although some 2 million women were exposed to DES in the womb, the number of reported cases of associated cancer is only slightly more than 400, a risk so slight that it can be ignored. A woman who knows that she is a DES daughter (and, as usual, the drug was marketed under many different and unedifying names, for example, Desplex, Benzestrol, and Estilben) should have a Pap smear every six to twelve months, but that's not a bad idea anyway.

Another substance that is almost surely not worth worrying about in the context of birth defects is TCDD—commonly called dioxin—the well-known contaminant in Agent Orange and the herbicide 2,4,5-T (a component of Agent Orange). TCDD is teratogenic and carcinogenic in animals and exposure to it causes the skin disease chloracne in humans. Repeated epidemiological studies in humans, however, in places as diverse as Arizona, Arkansas, Swedish Lapland, and New Zealand, have failed to show any association between 2,4,5-T and human birth defects.

Teratologists are fond of saying that every time a pregnant woman takes a drug (including alcohol, tobacco, and caffeine), she is performing an experiment in human teratology. An experiment of another sort began on Saturday, July 10, 1976, when a chemical plant making trichlorophenol exploded near Seveso, Italy, some 13 miles (20 kilometers) north of Milan. The result was that between 0.5 and 5 kilograms (kg) of TCDD (1–11 pounds) were deposited over several square miles of heavily populated countryside, along with much larger amounts of trichlorophenol and sodium hydroxide (caustic soda). Nearly 6,000 persons lived in an area that was contaminated with TCDD at levels from 1 microgram to 1 milligram per square meter.

These are astronomical amounts. The herbicide 2,4,5-T, as presently manufactured, contains about 10 micrograms of TCDD per kilogram. To kill brush, 2,4,5-T is applied at the rate of about 10 kilograms per 10,000 square meters; the resulting TCDD level is about one thousandth of a microgram per square meter. Exposures at Seveso were 1,000 to 1 million times higher than agricultural exposures.

What was the result in terms of birth defects of this enormous exposure to TCDD? In 1977, the year following the explosion, 2,756 children were born in Seveso; of these, 41 (1.5 percent) had frank malformations. In 1978, there were 90 obviously malformed children from 2,777 Seveso births, or 3.2 percent. This apparent increase is still within the normal malformation rate in western Europe, and the geographical distribution of birth defects in Seveso bears no relation to TCDD concentration.[19] So even this spectacular "experiment" provided no evidence that TCDD at very high levels is teratogenic to humans.

There is another danger, however, to which all women of child-bearing age should give some thought: fetal alcohol syndrome (FAS).

This problem was first recognized in the 1960s by the French scientists A. Giroud and H. Tuchman-Duplessis, and by P. Lemoine and his colleagues, and was emphasized in this country by P. L. Jones and his co-workers beginning in 1973. Children with FAS are, in varying degrees, both physically and mentally retarded. Their heads are small for their height, and they have minor anomalies of the face, eyes, joints, heart, and external genitalia.

Fewer than half the children of chronic alcoholic mothers (and possibly fathers) have FAS. But the important thing is that one needn't be a latter-day inhabitant of some Hogarthian Gin Lane to give birth to a child with FAS. *Daily* consumption of as little as 1 ounce of absolute (100 percent) alcohol significantly increases the risk. The approximate equivalent of an ounce of absolute alcohol is one dry Martini, two mixed drinks, or four (half-full) glasses of wine. The National Institute on Alcohol Abuse and Alcoholism concludes: "For baby's sake . . . and yours, don't drink during pregnancy."

This recommendation is controversial, but women who are pregnant or who are planning to become pregnant should confine themselves to a glass or two of wine or beer a day, with only occasional consumption of stronger drinks; or perhaps better yet, they should consider not drinking until their child is born. The authors of an article in the June 1982 issue of *Teratology* point out that when pregnant rats are given levels of alcohol in their diet that are like those produced by "social drinking," the cerebellar weights of the animals' brains are significantly reduced compared with controls, although the whole brain weights are the same in both groups.

Amniocentesis, in addition to its role in discovering genetically determined birth defects, can also be used to discover birth defects that can be repaired while the child is still in the womb. Nicole Whitmore, born in San Francisco early in 1981, was found by amniocentesis to have a rare disease that made her dependent on large quantities of the B vitamin biotin. Her older brother has the same disease and was lethargic or comatose and susceptible to infection before the nature of his illness was discovered. Nicole's mother, Debra Whitmore, was given large quantities of the vitamin beginning in the twenty-fourth week of her pregnancy, and Nicole arrived in the world as a healthy and normal baby. Like her brother, she must take biotin for the rest of her life, but she is otherwise completely normal.

Unfortunately, the March of Dimes National Foundation, which is now devoted to preventing birth defects, withdrew its support for amniocentesis because parents, knowing that their child will be born with a serious birth defect that will prevent it from ever living a normal life, may elect to have the damaged fetus aborted. Opposition to allowing parents to make this choice forced the National Foundation to cease encouraging amniocentesis. An interesting question may arise in the future as to whether a government that prohibits abortion can be sued by parents whose child is born with a major defect when, knowing that the child was defective, the parents might have chosen abortion.

Neural tube defects are among the most common major malformations (about 2 per 1,000 births) and can have tragic consequences. This group of defects includes spina bifida, in which a portion of the spinal cord protrudes from the vertebrae; exencephaly, in which only a rudimentary brain (or none at all) is present; encephalocele, in which the brain protrudes from an opening in the skull; and hydrocephalus, in which cerebrospinal fluid fails to drain normally from the ventricles of the brain, leading to a great increase in intracranial pressure that inhibits normal growth of the fetal and infant brain. The result of hydrocephalus is often severely reduced intelligence and dire physical handicaps. These defects seem to have a largely genetic basis and no environmental component, at least in Los Angeles County (*Teratology,* June 1982); there is a maternal age effect in spina bifida. In Los Angeles County between 1966 and 1972, more than half the exencephalic infants were stillborn and encephalocele was mercifully rare. The combined incidence of these two defects plus spina bifida (the commonest of the neural tube defects) was 1.1 per 1,000 births.

Neural tube defects can be detected with a high degree of confidence by a battery of tests. High levels of a substance (alpha-fetoprotein) appear in the mother's blood if the defect is present. Examination of the fetus by uterine sonography (ultrasound) permits localization of the defect, and its presence and location can be confirmed by X-ray or by the direct examination of the fetus *in utero* by fetoscopy, in which a fiber optic telescope is inserted directly into the uterus. Measurement of the nerve enzyme acetylcholine-esterase in maternal blood is also useful. None of these tests is adequate alone, but a battery of measurements gives a reliable diagnosis.

A child with exencephaly will either be stillborn or will die a day or two after birth. Occasionally, such an unfortunate child will live as long as a month. Spina bifida occurs in two forms. If the spinal cord is covered by skin, the defect can be surgically repaired and the child may survive with no, or only minor, physical problems. Only about one spina bifida victim in five is so lucky. In the majority of cases the spinal cord is exposed, and these children are generally retarded. They are also frequently paralyzed from the waist down, or have no bowel or bladder control in the absence of complete paralysis. Intensive treatment is required to keep them alive.

In the United Kingdom, tests for neural tube defects began being offered to pregnant women in 1974 and testing now includes nearly half the pregnant women in the population. When neural tube defects are detected, the women and their husbands are offered the choice between an abortion or letting nature take its course. Although the analysts of the U.S. Centers for Disease Control estimate that such a screening program would save at least two dollars for each dollar that it would cost, to say nothing of the reduction of human misery, the United States has been slow to adopt a screening program because of the opposition of right-wing extremists.

So much for the bad news. Some very good news is that neural tube defects may be prevented by vitamin supplementation of the diets of women planning a pregnancy, particularly those who have already borne such a child.[20] More good news is that hydrocephalus is now, and even spina bifida may ultimately be, treatable *in utero*. Drs. Marie Michejda and Gary Hodgen of the National Institute of Child Health and Human Development have developed a valve that can be surgically implanted in the fetal skulls of monkeys with hydrocephalus and set to release cerebrospinal fluid into the amniotic cavity when the intracranial pressure rises above a chosen point. The device has successfully prevented the symptoms of the disease in monkeys treated *in utero* with the valve and later delivered by Caesarean section.[21]

A similar approach has been applied to human fetuses with hydrocephalus by a University of Colorado School of Medicine team headed by Dr. William Clewell. The team consisted of three obstetricians, two radiologists with considerable experience in ultrasonic monitoring, a neurosurgeon, and a bioengineer with a D.Sc. degree. The group had had considerable experience implanting devices in the brains of newborns that had developed hydrocephalus postnatally. Some of the infants they had previously treated weighed less than one and a half pounds.

Then a twenty-six-year-old Arizona woman, twenty-one weeks pregnant with her third child, was examined by amniocentesis and ultrasound because of a family history of chromosome aberrations and a previously affected male child. Her baby was found to be developing hydrocephalus. Since she and her husband did not wish to terminate the pregnancy, they were referred to the Denver hospital Two weeks later, another ultrasound examination showed that the fetus's condition was worsening.

The medical team sought permission from the Medical Center's Human Subjects Committee to implant a shunt in the fetus's brain to dump excess fluid from the brain into the surrounding amniotic fluid. The fetus's parents could give informed consent for the mother, but who would be an advocate for the fetus? Ideally, it should be a neutral party standing, as it were, between the fetus and the physicians seeking to treat it. The Human Subjects committee appointed a theologian and a pediatrician specializing in care of the newborn (a neonatalogist) to act in this capacity.

On Wednesday, April 29, 1981, in the twenty-fourth week of gestation, an incision was made in the mother's abdomen under local anesthetic and the shunt was carefully inserted through a blunt needle that penetrated the fetal membranes, the amniotic fluid, and the fetal skull. After positioning the shunt, the needle was withdrawn so that the fetus could continue to move freely in its normal habitat.

The ventricles of the brain began immediately to return to normal dimensions, although complete normality was never achieved. For two months, everything worked smoothly. Then a strand of cells grew into the shunt and blocked passage of cerebrospinal fluid out of the brain. The child, who now weighed slightly more than five pounds in the eighth month of gestation, was promptly delivered by Caesarean section on July 16, 1981, and, after a period of stabilization, the intrauterine shunt was removed and the more usual type of postnatal shunt was installed in its place. The child went home after four weeks in the hospital.

At a little more than four months of age the infant boy, although small for his age and with repairable heart and other visceral abnormalities, was steadily improving. Of course, it will be years before it is clear to what extent normal physical and intellectual development has taken place. Since then two additional fetuses with hydrocephalus have been similarly treated *in utero* with this landmark procedure. All three infants appear to be much better off than if they had been allowed to go to term without intervention.

The NIH team of Michejda and Hodgen has also experimented with an agar-based medium containing bone powder that may be used as a paste while the baby is still in the womb to enclose the exposed spinal cord of a baby suffering from spina bifida in a sort of artificial vertebra that will at least protect the cord until more permanent repairs can be made following delivery.[22] Finally, Dr. Hodgen has found that if the fingers of monkeys are severed *in utero*, they can regenerate like so many starfish arms. This astonishing finding suggests the possibility that limb defects, and perhaps others, can be corrected *in utero* and the wounds healed before the infant is even delivered. If the shortened limbs of a thalidomide baby had been removed *in utero,* would they then have regenerated as normal babies since the teratogenic agent was no longer present? The prospects are tremendously exciting.

So, despite the fact that it is still true that there is no teratogen for humans or laboratory animals whose mode of action we completely understand, progress is being made that holds great hope for the future. A more disheartening aspect is the relative indifference to birth defect research that permeates much of the federal government, from which most research support ultimately comes. This indifference is awkward even when basic research is highly regarded. In periods like the present, it is catastrophic.

Finally, there is the Bendectin saga. Bendectin is sold by pre-scription only specifically to control the nausea and vomiting of pregnancy. In some quarters it is being hailed as "the new thalidomide," and currently the manufacturer faces from 36 to 200 lawsuits (depending on whose figures you choose to believe). As Bendectin has been on the market since 1956 and has been taken by some 30 million women, it is hardly new. So in what way does it resemble thalidomide and who says so?

Chemically, Bendectin bears no resemblance to thalid-omide. For the first twenty years of its existence, Bendectin was marketed as a mixture of 10 milligrams each of doxyla-mine succinate, pyridoxine hydrochloride, and dicyclomine hydrochloride. The last component, used in treating colic in infants since it relieves smooth muscle spasms in the gas-trointestinal tract, was removed from the mixture in 1976, since it increased the risk of complications without enhancing Bendectin's efficacy.

Doxylamine succinate is an antihistamine present in several over-the-counter preparations such as Vicks Formula 44 Cough Mix and Unisom Nighttime Sleep-Aid. There is no evidence that either doxylamine succinate or dicyclomine hydrochloride separately causes birth defects in animals, including man.

The third component of the original Bendectin, and one of the two remaining in the current form, is pyridoxine hydrochloride. Pyridoxine (and the closely related compounds into which it is transformed in the body) is better known as vitamin B_6, a substance required in the diet of all animals in very small amounts. One Bendectin tablet supplies five times the recommended daily allowance of pyridoxine, but an excess is not harmful. This is not true for the fat-soluble vitamins such as vitamin A, for example, which are teratogenic in great excess.

If Bendectin has the teratogenic properties of thalidomide, these properties must reside in the mixture of the three components available before 1977, since none of the individual components is known to be teratogenic.

Who says Bendectin is teratogenic? For its first twenty-one years on the market, nobody did. In fact, in February 1978, Dr. Richard Smithells, an English pediatrician and distinguished teratologist, and a co-worker, Dr. Sheila Sheppard, published a study of over 2,000 births from which they concluded: "We found no evidence to suggest that Bendectin is teratogenic to humans."[23] This was an important conclusion because an estimated 25 percent of pregnant women in America take the drug. Bendectin is seriously overprescribed. Only about 10 percent of pregnant women need such a drug to prevent the severe dehydration resulting from repeated vomiting that could require their hospitalization; Bendectin is the only prescription drug approved by FDA for this use.

In April 1979, Dr. Kenneth Rothman of Harvard and a group of colleagues from various Boston medical schools published a study on congenital heart defects in children. The authors pointed out very clearly that the "findings reported here . . . should be considered as no more than exploratory."[24] The findings were that Bendectin consumption had a weak association (in a small number of patients) with congenital heart disease. But stronger associations with congenital heart disease were obtained with a semisynthetic penicillin (Ampicillin), Valium, codeine, phenobarbital, and other common drugs, although in each case the number of patients available was limited. These small samples were a major reason for the authors' caution concerning their results.

The fervor over Bendectin was apparently sparked by an article in *The National Enquirer*, in October 1979. The Bendectin article was yellow journalism at its worst, complete with pictures of babies whose ghastly deformities were due— in *The Enquirer's* opinion—to their mothers having taken Bendectin.

One of the afflicted children pictured was David Mekdeci, five, of Orlando, Florida. David's deformed right hand was attached to a shortened right forearm. The pectoral muscles were missing from his right chest and his breastbone was also deformed. This constellation of malformations is the rare condition known as Poland syndrome (named for its discoverer). David's parents, Michael and Elizabeth Mekdeci, sued the manufacturer of Bendectin for $10 million in punitive damages and $2 million in compensatory damages.

The outcome of the trial seemed virtually certain. The Mekdecis' lawyer was the flamboyant Melvin Belli, who has since been advertising in U.S. papers for more cases of alleged Bendectin deformity. Belli imported Dr. William McBride— one of the discoverers of the teratogenicity of thalidomide in humans—from Sydney, Australia. Dr. McBride was well compensated. In addition to his travel and expenses, he was paid approximately $1,100 for each day that he was away from his obstetrical practice.

Yet another plus for Melvin Belli was the fact that Bendectin's manufacturer was none other than Richardson-Merrell, the firm that had attempted to import thalidomide into the United States and whose last "best-seller" in the 1960s, Mer-29, was forced off the market following an FDA raid on the firm. The raid produced evidence that the company had falsified the data it supplied to the government agency. Richardson-Merrell ultimately paid more than $2 million in damages in connection with Mer-29.

In addition, the jury of ordinary men and women was confronted with the unnerving spectacle of the cruelly deformed boy and the necessity of deciding who was to blame. If David had been struck by lightning, the question wouldn't have arisen. But when a deformed child is born there is, all too often, a frantic search for someone—parent, doctor, employer, or manufacturer—who can be blamed for the tragedy.

Incredibly, after hearing the evidence in January 1980, the Florida jury concluded that nothing should be awarded to David Mekdeci, and his parents were denied damages. The jury did, however, award $20,000 for medical expenses. This was a far cry from the $12 million the Mekdecis had sought; in May 1980, federal Judge Walter E. Hoffman ordered a retrial on the grounds that the jury's verdict was inconsistent. If the child was not damaged by Bendectin, as the jury had concluded, then the parents should recover nothing, he ruled. The retrial took nine weeks before a jury of five women and two men. They deliberated only two hours before reaching the verdict, on April 9, 1981, that Bendectin did not cause David Mekdeci's birth defects. Melvin Belli was not present. Describing Elizabeth Mekdeci as "A very difficult woman to work with," he had chosen not to represent the family at the retrial.[25]

Meanwhile, on Monday, September 15, 1980, an FDA panel met in a hot room crowded with lawyers and reporters to review the animal and human epidemiological data on Bendectin. Dr. McBride presented his views and Dr. Beverly Paigen, a cancer researcher (rather than a teratologist) at the Roswell Park Memorial Institute in Buffalo, New York, who has actively supported the idea that the malformations of children born to Love Canal parents were the result of their exposure to toxic chemicals, offered her opinion that Bendectin caused birth defects in 5 of every 1,000 women who took it. The FDA panel was not impressed.

Later in the two-day hearing, a number of experts discussed the thirteen studies available at that time that showed Bendectin to be at least as safe as any other drug and probably safer than most since it has been far more intensively studied. As one observer recalls: "The representatives of the press began to leave the room as soon as scientific testimony on Bendectin's lack of teratogenicity began to be given. It's a failure of the news media. They don't want to educate people about the causes of birth defects."[26]

This view was soon reinforced. In November 1980, the magazine *Mother Jones* had a four-page article on Bendectin that rivaled that of *The National Enquirer*. "A special *Mother Jones* investigation has revealed that reports . . . *suggest* that the drug *may* have caused thousands of Thalidomide-like birth defects in the children of women who took it" (italics added). To the careful reader, the many qualifiers indicated that *Mother Jones* had grave doubts about its own story (or at least the magazine's attorneys did), but that didn't stop them from printing it. And a pregnant woman who had been taking Bendectin had to wonder, after reading the story, if she should seek an abortion. In the opinion of Robert L. Brent, M.D., Ph.D., and a witness in over a hundred trials involving birth defects, hundreds of women who had taken Bendectin had healthy fetuses aborted because of the fear that their babies would be deformed.[27] In a real sense *The National Enquirer* and *Mother Jones* were accessories to the murders of healthy, wanted children.

On May 5, 1981, Jack Anderson took up the *National Enquirer–Mother Jones* line. A month later, the *Journal of the American Medical Association* published two articles, one from Boston University, the other from the Centers for Disease Control. The Boston group concluded that "early *in utero* exposure to Bendectin does not appreciably increase the risk of oral clefts [cleft lip or palate] or selected cardiac defects."[28] The CDC study of over 280,000 births concluded that "No associations were found between any of these [ten major] defect categories and Bendectin exposure."[29]

About the same time, I was making a survey of my own in Berlin. I asked five leading teratologists (from Britain, France, West Germany, Finland, and Israel) separately for their opinions about Bendectin. They were unanimous in proclaiming it as demonstrably safe as a drug could be. In the words of a reporter for *Science* magazine, "It remains the best studied drug taken by pregnant women."[30] Despite this, Ralph Nader's Health Research Group petitioned the Department of Health and Human Services on July 15, 1981, to remove Bendectin from the market.

It is impossible to say that Bendectin (or any other drug) is incapable of causing birth defects. Yet it is possible to say of Bendectin—as of few, if any, other drugs—that the risk of it causing a serious birth defect is 1 in 1,000 or less, possibly much less.

Meanwhile the lawsuits over birth defects go on and on. Most of them are lost. Even when they're won, the malformed child and its parents get only a fraction of every dollar of the settlement awarded after what are commonly years of litigation. The damage done to the lives of families caught up in these protracted legal battles is immense, and is quite possibly far more devastating to the family's continued healthy existence than was the initial birth of the handicapped child.

There are approximately 3.5 million children born each year in the United States. Conservatively, 2 percent, or 70,000, have a serious birth defect. This is a scientific, medical, legal, moral, and financial problem of stunning proportions and, although it doesn't seem to be getting any worse (in terms of the proportion of malformed children born), it is not improving very rapidly. Parents of such children, already the victims of a cruel turn of fate, risk being victimized again by attorneys anxious to rush them into years of litigation that, most often, leave them with no financial compensation for the corrosive effects of those years on the family's ability to adjust to its changed circumstances.

Case after futile case is brought to trial, only to be demolished by a few minutes' testimony of an experienced teratologist. One suggestion is that an impartial review board be created by an organization like the American Teratology Society to offer its professional opinion, as a friend of the court, as to whether the birth defect in question could reasonably have been caused by the event that the plaintiff (and the plaintiff's attorney) are claiming as the cause.[31]

It needs to be emphasized to the courts and to the legal profession that maternal psychological or physical trauma (as in an automobile accident) is an improbable cause of birth defects, as is the consumption of most drugs and even repeated exposure to diagnostic X-rays. (Radiation, therapeutic or otherwise, causes less than 1 percent of all birth defects.)[32] And there is nothing that happens during the period from conception to birth that causes hereditary defects or chromosomal aberrations like Down syndrome, for example. These facts alone would cause a great many suits to be terminated at an early stage and substantially reduce unnecessary suffering —although possibly lawyers' incomes would be reduced as well.

The contingency fee approach, so greatly admired by the *Times* (London) team that wrote the definitive story of thalidomide because it renders the courts of America accessible to everyone, has turned into a legal nightmare where it sometimes seems that everyone is suing everyone else. Possible solutions include routine legal insurance (analogous to medical insurance) and no-fault malpractice insurance with compulsory and binding arbitration.[33]

Although there is no epidemic of birth defects, lawsuits concerning them have attained epidemic proportions, and this legal epidemic has led to a corresponding epidemic increase in human misery and unnecessary suffering.

Epilogue

It's frustrating to come to the end of writing this book and—having hoped to cover so much—have finally done so little. There were so many stories I wished to share, but there was too little time and too little space.

Perhaps some of these stories can be part of another book, along with other scientific adventures that I've only just heard of, for new and important diseases turn up frequently, and our ignorance, about infectious disease particularly, seems much more impressive than our knowledge.

This book is a collection of stories about, in addition to birth defects and allegations of biological warfare, eight different diseases that are known to be—or probably are—microbial in origin; that is, caused by bacteria, viruses, or fungi. Two of these eight, botulism and Hansen's disease, have long been known to be of bacterial origin. Of the remaining six, five have been discovered within most of our lifetimes (that is, within the last twenty-five years) and another (swine flu) was thought to be a museum piece. Of the five "new" diseases, the agents of two (Reye syndrome and Kawasaki disease) remain unknown, and there are imposing mysteries still connected with Hansen's disease, Legionnaires' disease, botulism (particularly the infant form), Toxic Shock Syndrome, and genital herpes. Of these five diseases, moreover, only two (Legionnaires' disease and Toxic Shock Syndrome), are readily curable under favorable conditions.

Legionnaires' disease is the most numerically significant of the "new" life-threatening diseases (some 100,000 cases each year in the United States); it was discovered only in 1976. That same year infant botulism, by far the most prevalent form of the disease, was recognized for the first time. Legionnaires' disease accounts for about one eighth of the cases of atypical pneumonias that occur in the United States each year. The cause(s) for the remaining seven-eighths remain unknown. In this important area the extent of our ignorance is at least seven times greater than that of our knowledge.

Toxic Shock Syndrome associated with tampon use was first recognized in 1980. A dozen years ago genital herpes was a rarity. Today there are 300,000 new cases reported each year in the United States.

Looking back, then, the theme of this book has to be our profound ignorance, a hundred years after Pasteur, of the world of pathogenic—that is, illness-producing—microorganisms.

These facts emphasize the point so eloquently made by Lewis Thomas, M.D., in his book *The Medusa and the Snail*. He writes: "The only solid piece of scientific truth about which I feel totally confident is that we are profoundly ignorant about nature. Indeed, I regard this as the major discovery of the past one hundred years of biology. . . . It would have amazed the brightest minds of the eighteenth-century Enlightenment to be told by any of us how little we know and how bewildering seems the way ahead. It is this sudden confrontation with the depth and scope of ignorance that represents the most significant contribution of twentieth-

Notes

Chapter 1: Without the Camp

1. Graham Greene, *A Burnt-Out Case* (New York: Viking Press), pp. 19–20. Copyright © 1960, 1961, 1974 by Graham Greene. (Published in Great Britain by William Heinemann & The Bodley Head.)

2. T. M. Vogelsand, "Gerhard Henrik Armauer Hansen, His Life and His Work," *International Journal of Leprosy* 46:257 (1978).

3. Ibid., p. 228.

4. *Int. J. Leprosy* 43:45 (1975).

5. G. Armauer Hansen and Carl Looft, *Leprosy* (London: Simpkin, Marshall, Hamilton, Kent & Co. Ltd., 1895), p. 94.

6. *Int. J. Leprosy* 8:137 (1940).

7. Stanley Stein and Lawrence Blockman, *Alone No Longer*, by *The Star* (Carville, La., 1963, 1974), p. 37.

8. Ibid., p. 72.

9. *Science* 215:1083 (26 February 1982).

10. Ibid. See also *Journal of the American Medical Association* 247:2283 (1982).

11. *The Star* 40, No. 1, 7 (1980).

12. Interview, W. F. Kirchheimer, *The Star* 38, N. 6, 13 (1979).

13. See note 9.

14. *The Star* 40, No. 1, 6 (1980).

15. *Leviticus* 13:1–59.

16. *The Star* 40, No. 1, 2 (1980).

17. *The Star* 39, No. 1, 5 (1980).

18. NBC Evening News, October 14, 1976. Vanderbilt Television News Archives, Vanderbilt University, Nashville, Tenn.

Chapter 2: The Great Bicentennial Swine Flu Caper

1. Dr. Sencer's memo is reproduced in Richard E. Neustadt and Harvey Finegold, M.D., *The Swine Flu Affair* (Washington, D.C.: U.S. Government Printing Office, 1978), pp. 147–55.

2. Ibid., p. 156.

3. *Science* 192:636 (1976).

4. © CBS Inc. 1976. All rights reserved. Originally broadcast March 24, 1976, over the CBS television network on the CBS Evening News.

5. Transcript of the subcommittee hearing, pp. 7, 9.

6. *Congressional Record—House*, April 5, 1968, p. 9453.

7. Gerald R. Ford, *Public Papers of the Presidents*, Vol. II, 1976–77, pp. 1131–32.

8. See note 1, p. 33.

9. *Saturday Review*, November 27, 1976, p. 7.

10. *Science* 192:640 (1976).

11. See note 1, p. 39.

12. Ibid., p. 13.

13. *Science* 194:334 (1976).

14. *Nature* 260:381 (1976).

Chapter 3: The Perilous Voyage of the Good Ship NIP

1. *Business Week*, July 19, 1976, p. 27.

2. *New York Times*, June 16, 1976, 50:5.

3. Richard E. Neustadt and Harvey V. Finegold, M.D., *The Swine Flu Affair* (Washington, D.C.: U.S. Government Printing Office, 1978), p. 53.

4. Senate Reports, Nos. 717–769, 94th Congress, 2nd session, Report 742, p. 4.

5. See note 3, p. 53.

6. Ibid., p. 50.

7. Text of statement by Albert Sabin, M.D., prepared on June 28, 1976, for the Roger Subcommittee (kindly furnished by Dr. Sabin).

8. Dr. Sabin's statement, pp. 1–3; and *The Journal of Infectious Diseases* 134:100 (1976).

9. Copy of this letter kindly furnished by Dr. Sabin.

10. Edwin D. Kilbourne, "A $135 Million Gamble," in *Natural History*, June–July 1976, pp. 39.

11. *Science* 193:560 (1976).

12. Ibid.

13. See note 3, p. 29.

14. *New York Times*, August 4, 1976, 13:2.

15. Opening statement by Senator Kennedy, Subcommittee on Health of the Senate Committee on Labor and Public Welfare, August 5, 1976.

16. *Science* 193:1225 (1976).

17. Ibid., p. 1224.

18. From the copyrighted interview, "If Swine Flu Strikes—Why Medical Men Are Worried," in *U.S. News and World Report*, September 20, 1976, p. 28.

19. Ibid., p. 29.

20. *The New England Journal of Medicine* 295:759 (1976).

21. *Bulletin of the New York Academy of Medicine* 55:285 (1979).

22. *Science* 194:590, 648 (1976).

23. Ibid.

24. *American Journal of Law and Medicine* 3:426 (Winter 1977–78).

25. *Annals of Internal Medicine* 87:769 (1977).

26. See note 21.

27. See note 3, p. 67.

28. *New York Times*, October 16, 1976, 50:1.

29. See note 25.
30. Ibid.
31. *New York Times,* December 10, 1976, II, 7:5.
32. *Archives of Internal Medicine* 118:139 (1966).
33. *Journal of the American Medical Association* 240:1616 (1978).
34. *American Journal of Epidemiology* 110:105 (1979).
35. *New York Times,* March 28, 1977, p. 49.

Chapter 4: Toxic Shock

1. CBS Evening News, October 6, 1980. Vanderbilt Television News Archives, Vanderbilt University, Nashville, Tenn.
2. *New York Times,* August 18, 1980, III, 3:5.
3. *New York Times,* August 30, 1980, 14:5.
4. Associated Press, April 22, 1982.
5. *Science* 211:842 (1981).
6. *The Journal of Infectious Diseases* 143:509 (1981).
7. *The Lancet,* May 9, 1981, 1017.
8. *Morbidity and Mortality Weekly Report* 31:201 (1982).
9. *Journal of the American Medical Association* 247:1464 (1982).
10. Thomas Thompson, *Blood and Money,* Garden City, N.Y.: Doubleday and Co., 1978.

Chapter 5: Siberian Ulcer and Yellow Rain

1. Convention on the Prohibition of the Development, Production and Stockpiling of Bacteriological (Biological) and Toxin Weapons and Their Destruction.
2. Charles T. Gregg, *Plague!* (New York: Charles Scribner's Sons, 1978), p. 251.
3. *New York Times,* March 21, 1980, 1:6.
4. Ibid.
5. Ibid.

6. *New York Times,* March 21, 1980, 1:1.
7. *Nature* 284:294 (27 March 1980).
8. *New York Times,* March 29, 1980, 11:3.
9. *Science* 208:37 (4 April 1980).
10. *New York Times,* September 14, 1981, 1:5 ff.
11. *New York Times,* September 15, 1981, 1:1.
12. Ibid., 8:6.
13. New York: M. Evans and Co., 1981.
14. A. Z. Joffe, in S. Kadis, A. Ciegler, and S. J. Ajl, eds., *Microbial Toxins VIII, Algal and Fungal Toxins* (New York: Academic Press, 1971), p. 139.
15. *The Wall Street Journal,* December 30, 1981, p. 6.
16. *The Wall Street Journal,* November 6, 1981, p. 26.
17. See note 14.
18. United Press International, October 17, 1981.
19. Ibid., November 11, 1981.
20. *The Wall Street Journal,* December 30, 1981, p. 6.
21. *Time,* April 5, 1982, p. 26.
22. *Chemical and Engineering News,* February 1, 1982, p. 6.
23. United Press International, November 12, 1981.
24. See note 14.
25. *The Wall Street Journal,* April 28, 1982, p. 28.
26. A. Hoeber and J. Douglass, Jr., *International Security,* Summer 1978, p. 55.
27. *Science* 214:1008 (27 November 1981).
28. See note 26.
29. *Chemical and Engineering News,* November 16, 1981, p. 10.

Chapter 6: Slaughter of the Innocents

1. *Journal of the National Reye's Syndrome Foundation* 1, No. 2, 57 (1980).
2. *New Mexican,* February 26, 1980.
3. Ibid.
4. *Pediatrics* 60:708 (1977).
5. Ibid.
6. *Science* 207:1453 (1980).

7. *New York Times*, March 2, 1980, 21:1.

8. See note 1, p. 63.

9. See note 6.

10. *Canadian Medical Association Journal* 122:1013 (1980).

11. *Annual Review of Medicine* 33:569 (1982).

12. *Time*, August 25, 1980, p. 60.

13. *New England Journal of Medicine* 304:1568 (1981).

14. Personal communication from Col. David L. Huxsoll, Ph.D., and Maj. Gen. Garrison Rapmund, M.D., U.S. Army Medical Research and Development Command, Fort Detrick, Maryland, March 1982.

14. *The Lancet*, January 23, 1982, p. 191.

15. *Morbidity and Mortality Weekly Report* 31:53 (1982).

Chapter 7: Life and Death at the Bellevue Stratford

1. *New York Times*, August 6, 1976.

2. Ibid.

3. CBS Evening News, Vanderbilt University Television News Archives, Vanderbilt University, Nashville, Tenn.

4. *Family Health*, December 1976, p. 62.

5. *New York Times*, August 12, 1976, p. 28.

6. *Interview*, September 2, 1980.

7. *Science* 194:1027 (3 December 1976).

8. *New York Times*, October 7, 1977, p. 18.

9. *Journal of Infectious Diseases* 140:784 (November 1979).

10. *New York Times*, October 7, 1977, p. 18.

11. *New York Times*, January 15, 1979, II, p. 1.

12. *Newsweek*, September 18, 1978, p. 30.

13. Ibid.

14. *New York Times*, January 13, 1979, p. 25.

15. *Applied and Environmental Microbiology* 43:240 (1982).

16. Personal communication, Dr. Walter Dowdle, Director, Center for Infectious Disease, The Centers for Disease Control, May 10, 1982.

17. *Annals of Internal Medicine* 91:795 (1979).

Chapter 8: The Emperor's Sausage

1. *Albuquerque Journal*, July 2, 1978, p. A–1.
2. T. M. Pierce, *New Mexico Place Names* (Albuquerque: University of New Mexico Press, 1965), p. 37.
3. *Albuquerque Journal*, February 2, 1979, *Impact* section, p. 12.
4. Ibid., April 17, 1978, p. A–1.
5. Ibid., April 16, 1978, p. A–1.
6. Official Report on the Botulism Outbreak, Clovis, New Mexico, April 8–18, 1978. Health Services Division, State of New Mexico, July, 1978, part 1, p. 10.
7. See note 4.
8. *Albuquerque Journal*, April 29, 1978, p. B–3.
9. Ibid., April 20, 1978, p. B–16.
10. Ibid., June 13, 1978, p. A–3.
11. See note 6, part 3, p. 16.
12. *New York Times*, April 28, 1982, III, 1:1.
13. *Morbidity and Mortality Weekly* 31:87 (1982).
14. *The Journal of Pediatrics* 94:331 (1979).
15. *Annual Review of Medicine* 31:541 (1980).
16. *Epidemiologic Reviews* 3:45 (1981).
17. *American Journal of Public Health* 71:266 (1981).
18. See note 6, part 3, p. 19.

Chapter 9: A Virus of Love

1. Venereal disease is named for Venus, the Roman goddess of love. Half a dozen venereal diseases are caused by viruses, but they are either far less frequently encountered or less serious than herpes.
2. *Clinical Obstetrics and Gynecology* 15:896 (1972). *American Journal of Obstetrics and Gynecology* 133:548 (1979). *Western Journal of Medicine* 130:414 (1979).
3. *The New England Journal of Medicine* 304:759 (1981).
4. R. Hamilton, *The Herpes Book* (Los Angeles, J. P. Tarcher, Inc., 1980), p. 93.

5. See note 2.

6. *Morbidity and Mortality Weekly Report* 31:137 (1982).

7. *Annual Review of Medicine* 32:233 (1981).

8. *Annals of Neurology* 5:2 (1979).

9. See note 6, p. 98.

10. *Science* 181:161 (1973).

11. *The Lancet*, October 10, 1981, p. 777.

12. *The New England Journal of Medicine* 306:343 (1982); *The Lancet*, February 20, 1982, p. 421.

13. *Ebony*, June 1981, p. 42. Reprinted by permission of *Ebony* Magazine. © 1981 by Johnson Publishing Co., Inc.

Chapter 10: O Hateful Error, Melancholy's Child

1. *Suffer the Children: The Story of Thalidomide*, New York: Viking Press, 1978, p. 30.

2. Ibid., pp. 42–43.

3. Ibid., p. 75.

4. James G. Wilson and F. Clarke Fraser, eds., *Handbook of Teratology* (New York: Plenum Press, 1977), Vol. 1, p. 4.

5. Ibid., p. 75.

6. *Environmental Science and Technology* 15:626 (1981).

7. Christopher Norwood, *At Highest Risk* (New York: McGraw-Hill, 1980), pp. 29 ff.

8. *Morbidity and Mortality Weekly Report* 28:402 (1979).

9. See note 7.

10. *American Journal of Epidemiology* 114:548 (1981).

11. *Teratology* 21:323 (1980).

12. Michael Brown, *Laying Waste* (New York: Pantheon, 1979), p. 329.

13. *Journal of the National Cancer Institute* 66:1193 (1981).

14. Ibid.

15. *Science* 212:1404 (1981).

16. See note 1, p. 8.

7. *Journal of the American Medical Association* 246:758 (1981).

18. *Morbidity and Mortality Weekly Report* 30:38 (1981).

19. *Nature* 280:184 (1979).

20. *The Lancet*, January 30, 1982, p. 275.

21. See note 17, p. 1079.

22. Ibid., p. 1093.

23. *Teratology* 17:31 (1978).

24. *American Journal of Epidemiology* 109:433 (1979).

25. *Science* 210:518 (1980).

26. Robert L. Brent, Twenty-first Annual Meeting of the Teratology Society, Thursday, June 25, 1981.

27. See note 25.

28. *Journal of the American Medical Association* 245:2311 (1981).

29. See note 25, p. 2307.

30. See note 24.

31. *Journal of Pediatrics* 71:288 (1967).

32. James G. Wilson, in *Handbook of Teratology*, Vol. 1, 1977, p. 310.

33. *Teratology* 16:1 (1977).

Epilogue

1. Lewis Thomas, *The Medusa and The Snail: More Notes of a Biology Watcher* (New York: Viking Press, 1977), p. 73.

Index